"Gonzalez-Dolginko has given us a window into the historical, research, and theoretical antecedents of the Kestenberg Art Profile (KAP) that is introduced in this volume. The depth and breadth of this body of work integrating theory into clinical practice throughout the lifespan is clearly palpable throughout the book. This volume vividly illuminates clinical art therapy examples throughout the life cycle depicting how developmental art and movement can be expressed, understood, and then transformed."

—Susan Loman

"*Applying Developmental Art Theory in Art Therapy Treatment and Interventions* illuminates Dr. Beth Gonzalez-Dolginko's decades of first-hand experience (as a clinician, researcher, and parent) with human development as a valuable lens on which to practice creative arts therapy. Written in a down-to-earth, witty, and accessible narrative, Gonzalez-Dolginko's text will introduce a new generation of art therapists to the seminal theories of human development that support and help explain the potency of their work. She reminds readers of some of the most bedrock ideas of our profession that too few art therapists know about. This is a valuable book."

—Lynn Kapitan

Applying Developmental Art Theory in Art Therapy Treatment and Interventions

Illustrative Examples through the Life Cycle

Applying Developmental Art Theory in Art Therapy Treatment and Interventions: Illustrative Examples through the Life Cycle weaves clinical applications of object relations-based art therapy with the Kestenberg Art Profile to understand art from a developmental perspective with the intent of applying this knowledge to support best art therapy practice.

The book starts by defining object relations-based art therapy and introducing the Kestenberg Art Profile. Chapters blend psychological theory (Freud, Erikson, Piaget) and developmental art theory (DiLeo, Gardner, Kellogg, Levick, Lowenfeld and Brittain, and Rubin) with case illustrations that offer a focus on applying typical developmental theory and art therapy with children, adolescents, and adults who have varying needs. Examples include art from people throughout the life cycle with histories of trauma in the following areas: sexual, physical, and emotional abuse, terrorism, grief and medical illness, war, natural disasters, and substance abuse. There is further discussion on neurological indicators, family issues, and the use of materials and techniques viewed through a developmental lens.

Ideal for creative arts therapists, educators, and students, the book will also stand out as a supplementary text for developmental theorists and educators, art educators, and a range of mental health professionals.

Beth Gonzalez-Dolginko has worked clinically as an art therapist in institutions and private practice for over 40 years. Beth's specialty is human development. She has worked with children, adolescents, and adults.

Applying Developmental Art Theory in Art Therapy Treatment and Interventions

Illustrative Examples through the
Life Cycle

Beth Gonzalez-Dolginko

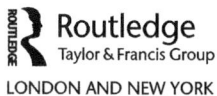

Routledge
Taylor & Francis Group

LONDON AND NEW YORK

First published 2022
by Routledge
2 Park Square, Milton Park, Abingdon, Oxon OX14 4RN

and by Routledge
52 Vanderbilt Avenue, New York, NY 10017

Routledge is an imprint of the Taylor & Francis Group, an informa business

© 2022 Beth Gonzalez-Dolginko

British Library Cataloguing-in-Publication Data
A catalogue record for this book is available from the British Library

Library of Congress Cataloging-in-Publication Data
Names: Gonzalez-Dolginko, Beth, author.
Title: Applying developmental art theory in art therapy treatment
and interventions: illustrative examples through the life cycle /
Beth Gonzalez-Dolginko.
Description: Abingdon, Oxon; New York, NY: Routledge, 2021. |
Includes bibliographical references and index. |
Summary: "This text weaves clinical applications of object relations-
based art therapy with the Kestenberg Art Profile to depict art
from a developmental perspective with the intent of applying this
knowledge to support best art therapy practice. Through examples
of developmental art theorists' contributions, case illustrations offer
a focus on the use of art therapy with children who have varying
needs including emotional disturbance, developmental delay or
social adjustment needs due to genetic or environmental factors,
developmental or learning disabilities, neurological impairment,
physical disabilities, cultural disadvantage, sexual and/or physical
abuse, severe trauma or medical illness"– Provided by publisher.
Identifiers: LCCN 2020055156 (print) | LCCN 2020055157 (ebook) |
ISBN 9780367858971 (paperback) | ISBN 9780367858988 (hardback) |
ISBN 9781003015611 (ebook)
Subjects: LCSH: Art therapy for children. | Kestenberg Movement Profile.
Classification: LCC RJ505.A7 G66 2021 (print) |
LCC RJ505.A7 (ebook) | DDC 618.92/891656–dc23
LC record available at https://lccn.loc.gov/2020055156
LC ebook record available at https://lccn.loc.gov/2020055157

ISBN: 978-0-367-85898-8 (hbk)
ISBN: 978-0-367-85897-1 (pbk)
ISBN: 978-1-003-01561-1 (ebk)

Typeset in Bembo
by Newgen Publishing UK

Contents

This book is dedicated to my mentors:
Judith Kestenberg
Arthur Robbins and
Michael Eigen
all of whom stoked the fires of my passion for
human development
and
to my grandsons, Ewan and Penn, who let me joyfully
watch development unfolding again

Preface

Welcome to my opus. This is a book that I have been writing in my head since my very first internship as an art therapy student. I interned and was then hired at a New York State facility for adults with developmental disabilities. Many of the residents additionally had mental illness and neurological complications. I did art therapy with them and collected artwork for five years. It was fascinating to me to observe developmental indicators in their art along with their behavior and social emotional development and to compare all of this to typical development.

As I continued in my career as an art therapist, became a professor, a psychoanalyst, and a mother, my fascination with human development and developmental art continued. Typical human development and developmental art is my research and what I taught. My hypothesis is that by viewing art through a developmental lens and by understanding typical developmental theory, a therapist's treatment and interventions in clinical practice will be more specific and effective with patients. Applying this knowledge supports best art therapy practice.

It is my great pleasure to introduce the Kestenberg Art Profile which examines and categorizes the art of infants and toddlers offering an additional method for understanding art developmentally. There are dozens of illustrative cases that offer a focus on applying a developmental perspective in art therapy with children, adolescents, and adults who have varying needs. Examples include art from people throughout the life cycle with histories of trauma in the following areas: sexual, physical, and emotional abuse, terrorism, grief and medical illness, war, natural disasters, and substance abuse. There is further discussion on applying this theory regarding neurological indicators, family issues, and the use of materials and techniques. I present to you decades of my work and research.

1 Introduction

This book is my life's work. The theory that informs my practice is object relations development. But I have to say that this is also my life's work because I have been interested in babies since I was a baby. At two, I would just watch my baby sister sleep because she was so cute. Sometimes, I awakened her, much to my mother's dismay, because she was *my* baby, and I wanted to play with her. My aunts loved me because I would entertain all babies and little kids at family parties, and they could just have fun. My Aunt Alice's sister-in-law ultimately had 15 children, but when I was the babysitting niece, she probably had seven or eight. My Aunt set up a corner in her basement, put down an area rug, and had a little rocking chair for me, along with other equipment needed to take care of infants and toddlers. I was in heaven, as I rocked a baby in my arms, another in a baby rocker with my foot, and read stories to toddlers. My older sisters and cousin, grateful to be relieved of the charge, supplied me with soda and snacks before they went off giggling to have teenager fun together.

As a tween and teen, I developed a significant babysitting practice that lasted till I left for college. And in college, I continued my interest in development through my studies and work in the college's Child Study Center. What I realized through my studies and observations was that, yes, I loved playing with, rocking, feeding, cooing with babies, but I was truly fascinated by observing their development. Raising my own children, and now as I babysit my grandsons, I delight at a baby finally grabbing a toy and then chewing on it, or finally defying gravity by getting a baby belly off the floor in preparation for crawling. And I relish all the milestones as life proceeds— saying words then sentences, reading a sentence, making the swing work in the playground without a grownup, and every other wonderful moment that unfolds at each stage.

In my own professional development, this natural fascination continued. I have always applied developmental theory to how I understood and made sense of patient art, made interpretations, and chose materials. And I taught all of this to art therapy students for decades. My own art therapy professors and supervisors, Arthur Robbins, Josef Garai, and Robert Wolf, were also psychoanalysts. The art therapy theory they offered wove psychoanalytic theory with paradigms for understanding the creative process. Object relations theory emerged significantly in their teachings as it was a good fit for studying the creative process in the transference and countertransference—the dance, the art object, the poem—as it develops between therapist and patient. I continued onto post-graduate psychoanalytic studies, focusing on object relations and attachment theory. One of my psychoanalytic professors, Michael Eigen, gave the best advice I ever got. He would tell us to look at the patient before us and imagine what kind of baby they were. Then, you have some insight into their development and know how to proceed with treatment. For example, if they are tightly strung and complain a lot, they may have been a whiny baby who had trouble getting their needs met. As the analyst, one frames interpretations so that the patient feels heard and held—what they did not feel as a baby.

My first art therapy job was in an inter-community facility (ICF) for adults with developmental disabilities. Most of the patients with whom I worked had resided in large state institutions; a small number came from family homes. ICFs were established to be a transitional residential and treatment facility for persons with developmental disabilities who previously resided in large state institutions, most of them for their entire lives. The goal was to eventually transition them back into the community. My work in the ICF gave me an opportunity to observe and study human development that occurred atypically. It spurred my belief in and research into theories of human development. To me, it was fascinating to see how the human spirit may be damaged by the environment yet transcends. I worked along with other creative arts therapists, and we all worked towards nurturing and healing that human spirit in our patients.

Life continued to bring me on a developmental path directly to Dr. Judith Kestenberg, internationally renowned child psychiatrist and psychoanalyst. One of my graduate art therapy students was doing her internship at Dr. Kestenberg's Child Development Research Center, and I made a site visit to observe the student in the setting. I was pregnant at the time with my first child (I am blessed to have four). Before Dr. Kestenberg even said hello, she looked at me and remarked, "You are a pregnant art therapist. You will come to my Center with your baby and supervise art therapy interns." I quickly learned that one does not say no to Dr. Kestenberg, and thus began a ten-year residency with a scholarly, and inimitable mentor.

My studies with Dr. Kestenberg and my chance to observe my own children's development galvanized my belief in and respect for this process, and I continued my application of this knowledge base to my clinical work. I must admit that I was put off by many of the client-centered psychological and counseling theories that were being taught in graduate therapy and counseling education programs in the 1980s. The emphasis is on what is going on right now in one's life and often dismisses the history that the patient brings to the treatment. The client would feel acceptance by the therapist, this would reflect back to them, and they would be able to move forward. I concede that many people want help with what is going on in their lives right then and there. Also conceded, people are less patient with or tolerant of long and drawn-out therapy and psychoanalytic relationships. Finally, the medical treatment model for behavioral health became short term, and treatment interventions were adjusted accordingly, calling for therapists to think about their work getting done in a constricted window of time.

Although I was only about a decade into my career at the time that this all occurred, I felt that the dismissal of a patient's history would interfere with their ability to satisfactorily resolve whatever it is that is going on in life for which they entered treatment. How can we help a patient move forward without looking at where they came from? Again conceded, we therapists had to do this in less time, but it was still necessary. Assessing the *baby* before us and understanding this baby's art presented in the session offers art therapists a way to get to some history quickly at the beginning of treatment. These observations and knowledge will inform the course of treatment and interventions.

As I offer the above advice to my students, I also urge them to study and learn what is typical in human development and developmental art. If we do not understand what is typical, we will not be able to truly see what is atypical. The ability to see what is atypical and understand where this occurred or stagnated along the developmental continuum gives us the knowledge needed to intervene effectively and efficiently. My studies of human development and developmental art are extensive and span over 46 years. Every time I observe this unfolding of human growth and development, I am filled with awe and respect. With an understanding of typical human development, an art therapist can make good decisions on how to proceed in treatment, concerning which materials to offer, framing interventions and interpretations, and recognizing developmental issues presented through the art.

Winnicott (1971b) once mused that psychoanalysis with children should not be a lengthy treatment process because children do not have years of neuroses piled onto developmental issues; therefore, he whimsically suggested that everyone should enter psychoanalysis as a child. We can conclude that it is more difficult to uncover years of neuroses and applying developmental theory to a patient's history gives us better tools for digging. This is my main hypothesis. I apply this knowledge in my work with people of all ages. Not only with children, but rather as the book title suggests throughout the life cycle.

Even as I write this book, a whole new world is emerging. We are dealing with a pandemic and lockdown. Families are sheltered-at-home with each other—schooling, working, exercising, recreating, cooking, and eating—as a unit, a closed set. As I share my observations of the last 46 years regarding the art of typically developing children, I realize that a few years from now, children's art may be different because of the pandemic. They may draw people with masks. That is what they are seeing when they go outside of their homes. There may be more fear represented in their eyes and facial expressions. As I walked to my car recently through two other parked cars in a parking lot, a little boy, who was sitting in the back seat with the windows opened, recoiled as I passed by, as if afraid of contact with me. This saddened me, but I realized this was our new normal.

I have seen changes in the art of children who are typically developing over the years. Social media and instant communication have affected children and adolescent art significantly, and more research is needed on this impact. One big change in children's artmaking happened when multicultural crayons were introduced. Previously, my observation was that most children did not color in faces of people they drew. Very simply, it is difficult to color in a face and try not to color over the eyes, nose, and mouth. But then, unless the features were adeptly drawn to represent an ethnicity, human figure drawings looked Caucasian. I observed that many children still did not color in faces, except children who were more gifted artists, but they had the colors from the multicultural crayons to fill in arms and legs, which supports their cultural identity.

Honestly, faces can be hard to draw. Most kids like to draw eyes, but noses are hard, and mouths, often showing emotion or mood, can be tricky. As I say many times in this book, most people stop drawing in early adolescence. The influence of Anime was significant and probably prolonged children's tolerance for drawing because it offered a stylized way to successfully draw faces. I am making a prediction. Young adolescents may continue to draw faces past their previous deadline to do so because they can now draw faces with masks on, thus avoiding the challenging rendering of the nose, mouth, and facial expression. In fact, masks have become a new opportunity to express personal creativity for everyone. One of my preadolescent patients wears a different mask each session from popsicles to tie-dye to hearts and flowers. All around me, I see masks that feature animal prints, batik, sports teams, big lips, and more whimsy. Perhaps this chance for people to make a creative statement is one of the good things that will come out of this pandemic.

Other changes were not so benign but are noteworthy. Trauma brings change to one's life and is reflected in the art of children who are typically developing. Being diagnosed with a medical illness or losing a loved one will certainly change the art of children who are typically developing.

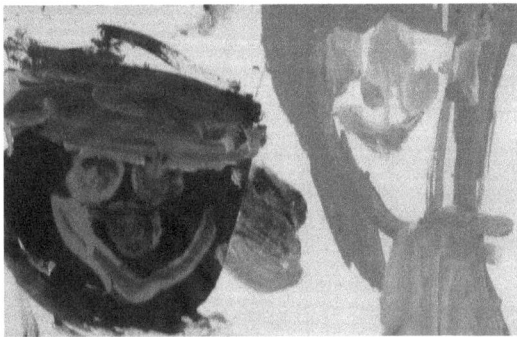

Figure 1.1 Drawing from a child who lost both parents to AIDS

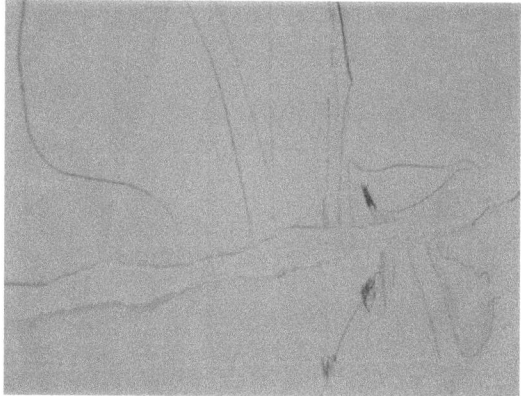

Figure 1.2 Drawing from a child who experienced an earthquake

More extreme circumstances, which impact our communities and societies, such as a natural disaster or terrorist attacks, result in changes in the art of children who are typically developing. And I am assuming that the COVID-19 pandemic and lockdown will also result in changes in the art of children who are typically developing. This remains to be seen. Therefore, I offer decades of observing children and their art as a foundation for working using a developmental art approach to the art therapy treatment process.

Reviewing artwork with an educated understanding of the stages of typical human development and typical art development will ensure that a clinician has a full picture of the patient regarding how to begin and engage in effective creative arts therapy treatment and result in good outcomes. The typical developmental art stages occur along with physical, psychosexual (Freud, 1905), psychosocial (Erikson, 1950), and cognitive (Piaget, 1936) stages of development and will be presented that way. Margaret Mahler and Judith Kestenberg have also contributed greatly to our understanding of early human development, and their theories are included. Using all these lenses gives us a clear picture. Looking at every aspect of the whole developing typical human being, from birth to death, is essential for a psychotherapist to do because without a deep knowledge of typical development, it is impossible to truly recognize and treat patients whose paths have not been typical.

In this book, I define object relations-based art therapy and have the distinct pleasure of introducing the Kestenberg Art Profile, both with illustrated examples. Theories of typical human development and art development are reviewed with illustrated examples from: infancy and early childhood; childhood; preadolescence; adolescence; and adulthood. Human development theorists included are Freud, Erikson, Piaget, and Kestenberg. Developmental art theorists included are Kestenberg (the Kestenberg Art Profile is introduced herein), Joseph H. DiLeo (1970, 1973, 1977, 1983),

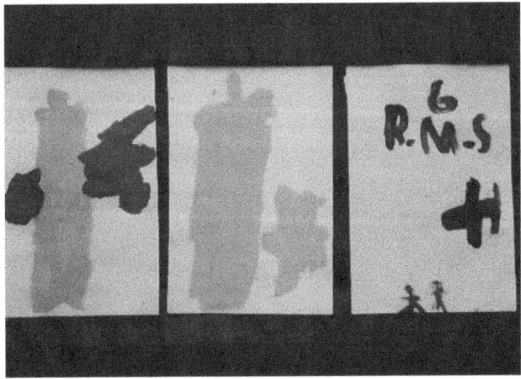

Figure 1.3 Drawing from a child who experienced the terror attacks of 9/11/01

Howard Gardner (1980), Rhoda Kellogg (1967), Myra Levick (1998), Viktor Lowenfeld and W.L. Brittain (1957), and Judith Rubin (1984).

Some art therapy assessments are reviewed throughout with examples, such as the *Silver Test of Cognitive and Creative Skills* (related to neurological indicators in the art), and the *Kinetic Family Drawing* (Burns and Kaufman, 1972). There is an exploration of age-appropriate and developmentally appropriate materials and techniques for use in treatment and interventions.

Life has many bumps in the road, and some result in challenges and trauma. This book contains research, theory, and clinical examples of the impact on human development due to physical differences, medical illness, and mental illness. Further included is significant research, theory, and clinical examples regarding trauma caused by physical, sexual, emotional abuse, grief and medical illness, substance abuse, and of severe trauma, related to disasters, war, and terrorism.

Please read on and enjoy and learn from my decades of research about human development and developmental art.

2 Object Relations and Art Therapy
Understanding the Theory

In Freud's later writings, he expanded the understanding of the human psyche to include interpersonal relations rather than simply intrapsychic dynamics. This resulted in the shift from the innate drive theory to understanding the value of primary relationships. The school of ego psychology rose out of the structural model of psychoanalysis (Freud, S., 1923) and defined distinct functions of the ego, the temporary absence of which indicates the presence of psychopathology. Object relations is one of the functions of the ego (Freud, A., 1937). It is the function of the ego that represents the ego's ability to attach to the object. The development of this function occurs in the first years of life.

Object Relations Based Creative Arts Therapy

Object relations based creative arts therapy supports the construction of the external object for the intention of better understanding the internalized object and its relation to a patient's ego development and attachment and separation issues for purposes of incorporating effective interventions into the treatment process. Object relations is a function of an organized ego, or self, that represents the person's ability to attach and connect with another person in a genuine and intimate way. In simple, developmental terms, the self is the baby, and the object is the mother. In a healthy mother and baby relationship, the infant develops a sense of body and mind *self* by a strong attachment to the mother, followed by a dance between mother and baby within that attachment, leading to the baby's ability to separate from the object with an internalized sense of self and object.

Many object relations theorists have given us language that easily translates into creative arts therapy theory and practice. Melanie Klein gave us a way to understand the formations of the infant's internal fantasies. In her work with children, she determined these fantasies grew out of the dynamic relationship (Klein, 1957) as opposed to an attempt to reduce the tension experienced by the internal drives when not gratified. The latter was the more common view of the British School of Psychoanalysis during the 1930s and the 1940s. Klein expanded on the infant fantasies and described the good breast and the bad breast (Mitchell, 1986). The good breast gives milk and the bad breast does not and frustrates. Klein hypothesized that love and trust grow out of the infant's capacity to both integrate and successfully split the loved and hated primal object.

While we may never know the infant's actual inner thoughts and dialogue, Klein is describing the infant's perception and experience of the object and the nature of this primary relationship. This useful imagery informs creative arts therapists' ability to understand the theory of object relations and its application to clinical practice.

In continuing with understanding the baby's fantasies, Eigen (1980) argues that it is not the breast, but rather the image of the object's face which the baby conjures up in the absence of the object, or mother.

> For the infant the appearance of the face is an indicator that another per-sonality is present. When the child is panicked at the mother's absence it is likely that an image of her face, not her breast, brings more comfort.
>
> (p. 439)

Spitz (1955) describes the child's image as their view of the mother's face and the reflection of self in the mother's eye. All of this enables us to under-stand the beautiful play that occurs in the baby's creative mind while looking into the mother's face in her presence and being able to remember her image in her absence.

Perhaps the object relations theorist that speaks most clearly to artists and therapists is D. W. Winnicott, who is one of the most understandable of the object relations theorists. Winnicott (1953) depicted imagery in three ways to observe the space between the self and the object: *Transitional Space, Intermediate Area of Experience*, and *Transitional Object*.

Winnicott defined the *Transitional Space* as the place where the external object begins to emerge. He defined the *Intermediate Area of Experience* as the space where the child plays and creates images of objects. There is no clear distinction between inner and outer reality in this space. The *Transitional Object* is an external object that allows a bridge between self and other, self and object, and supports the ego's ability to become separate. It relates back-wards in time to autoerotic phenomena and fist and thumb sucking and forward in time to attaching to the first external inanimate object. These are the earliest experiences of the healthy infant as expressed principally in the relationship between self and other and to the first possession—transitional object—or the first soft animal or doll, which relates both to the external object (mother's breast) and to internal objects (magically introjected breast), but is distinct from each. Gradually, the transitional object becomes decathected, sometimes as the infant develops and sometimes as external pressure is applied by caretakers.

The transitional objects and transitional phenomena belong to the realm of illusion made possible by the mother's special capacity for making adapta-tion to the needs of her infant, thus allowing the infant the illusion that what the infant creates really exists. To go further with this, there is a sense that the baby is then able to associate positive and fulfilling feelings to this illusion, hence allowing for the emergence of further images as representations of both inner and outer experiences. Creative arts therapists can be excited about this theory because it gives them insight into the evolution of one's image repertoire and the internal dialogue that thus ensues from the recollection of this image. It is remarkable to witness how one can recall a pre-verbal image during an art therapy session and then work towards understanding the significance.

Harold Searles (1979) observed toys or blankets that his patients brought to sessions and felt these reflected on the patient's ego development. He felt that inanimate objects became bridges between us and living objects, and they support us so that we can mirror and attune to those living objects. We project ourselves onto the inanimate object and transform them into intermediate objects that are the bridges to our first love. Robert Landy (1994) articulated the theory of role playing, used by drama therapists internationally. He described the development of *Role*, or ego, in humans. The fetus's role is to survive in an environment that provides a complete means of survival. The newborn's role is to adapt to a new, accommodating environment to survive, and in so doing, begins the separation between "me" and "not-me." Landy goes on to elaborate that the taking on of *Role* by humans leads to social constructs. A good adaptation to *Role* will support the person's ability to accommodate social constructs as they develop.

Space and Shape

Intrinsic to the relationship between self and object is the existence of the space in which fantasy emerges and play takes place. Let us look further into the concept of space and the representation of this in play and in art. Winnicott (1953) described the intermediate area of experience in which there is no clear distinction between the inner and outer reality—where the child plays and creates images of objects. The same area is also referred to as potential space between mother and child, a hypothetical area which exists and does not exist. Deri (1978) pointed out that in this creative area there is room for knowledge of the nature of real objects, not only for the sake of the reality principle but also for the recognition of the quality of the raw material out of which one creates. Deri thought that the transitional space is interwoven seamlessly with actual reality. In other words, it can be lifted out for the purpose of conceptualization. In Bergman's (1978) study of the actual space between mother and child, she distinguished between the actual and transitional space and referred to objects such as windows, doors, and vehicles as transitional spaces.

Perhaps the conceptualization of objects as space can be better understood by looking at what Boenig (1976) calls transitional ambiance. He describes a psychological rebirth that we all go through daily upon going from the state of sleep to being awake. Within the space which we have created around ourselves, we are able to reconstitute into the individual that we are as separate and differentiated from all others. In visual, tactile, and kinesthetic ways, we recreate around us that potential or transitional space that originally existed between self and other. Without this reorganization process, we will tend to feel lost in space, so to speak, and uncomfortable in the proceedings of our daily routine. The objects around us, of our own choosing, are therefore integral to this concept of space.

A possible source of confusion is created by the customary use of the phrase *inner space* as a metaphor denoting the location of psychic events. One easily forgets that in addition to the real outer space, there is also an inner space, as for instance the space in the mouth and in the lungs and other parts of the inside of the body. Spitz (1955) describes this space as the primal cavity. The multiplicity of terminology and definitions may stem from the fact we are dealing with an intermediate area of experience in which external reality is endowed with illusion. But this is indeed our concept of reality. There is no way we can really see what it is with the sense equipment available to us. We conclude as to the nature of reality, but we can hardly experience it concretely. Each of our senses can be used to explore through sight, sounds, touch, smell, and kinesthesis. However, final construction of the objects thus explored is based on an integration of the sensory motor experiences into a concept that belongs to our psychic life.

The conceptualization of objects as space is difficult to understand unless one thinks of the space taken up by the object, which is usually referred to as shape (Kestenberg, 1967; Kestenberg & Sossin, 1979). Shape is created by the meaning it receives from the baby's forming it into spatial configurations (Laban, 1966; Langer, 1954). Without objects, space is only a construct.

Along with the Sands Point Movement Study Group, Judith Kestenberg et al. (1971) developed the Kestenberg Movement Profile (KMP), which is used internationally by dance/movement therapists. The KMP assigns meaning to the infant's movements as the baby goes through attachment and separation. The shape and flow of the movement creates an external object, experienced on a body level, so that the baby can eventually make a healthy separation with a strong ego. This book introduces the Kestenberg Art Profile (KAP) in Chapter 3, which can be used to review the art products of young infants and toddlers and study the ways in which limited flat space can be utilized to create objects in space and how these objects give meaning to space by animating it.

Many creative arts therapists are familiar with Langer's (1954) term virtual space, an abstract concept on which visual art is based. Is virtual space available from the start? Does it have to develop and if so, how? How does virtual space differ from intermediate, transitional, potential, and actual aspects of space that are a part of what is essentially virtual space in art?

Langer's (1954) concept of virtual space in art is described as:

>...the harmoniously organized space in a picture is not experimental space, known by sight and touch, by free motion restraint, far and near

sounds, voices lost or re-echoed. It is an entirely visual affair; for touch and hearing and muscular action, it does not exist…and this purely visual space is an illusion, for our sensory experiences do not agree on it in their report…without the organizing shapes, it is simply not there. Like the space behind the surface of a mirror, it is what physicists call "virtual space, an intangible image."

(p. 71)

Langer goes on to say that virtual space is the primary illusion of all plastic art, and being only visual, this space has no continuity with the space in which we live. It is limited by the frame, which, however, does not really divide it from practical space. And then she seems to contradict herself when she points out that all boundaries not only separate but connect as well. Many creative arts therapists would disagree with her thesis that visual space does not exist without shape. Space and shape exist together.

Winnicott (1971a) expands on his term, *Intermediate Area of Experience*, and refers to a quality of space in which concepts of actual and illusory reality merge. It is not yet active as space. When Winnicott speaks of potential space between mother and child, he is describing an aspect of space which is created by the distance and the configuration of the space separating them. The transitional aspect of space is another way to define mergers between what appears to be real and illusory. The concept of space must be abstract, but the degrees and qualities of the abstraction change in development. Unchallenged in respect to its belonging to inner or external reality, Winnicott suggests that the intermediate area of experience constitutes the greater part of the infant's experience, and he feels it is retained throughout life in the intense experiencing that belongs to the arts, religion, and imaginative living—creativity.

A baby turns their head to reach the mother's nipple, through practice, and develops an idea that they must move for touch to occur. The baby may remember the feeling of touch and the feeling of non-touch, but there is a distinction between an actual sensory experience and its memory. Anna Freud (1944) thought that the baby has hallucinatory experiences of the maternal breast. Is this the nature of first memories, out of which the absence of the object and its existence in the past is differentiated from the global experience of perceiving what is not actually there?

The self-touch, be it one's hand on the surface of the body or one's hand into the mouth inside the body, brings with it the experience of being alive, being me. Projecting ourselves into space, we create new "me's" in the space. These new "me's" become the basis for the "not-me's" of the objects other than ourselves. We are back in Winnicott's (1971a) intermediate area in which the "me" and the "not-me" merge and unmerge. The further away the object, and especially when it is out of reach, the stranger it is and the less we can endow it with our own characteristics.

Let us now look at Piaget and Inhelder (1948) for cognitive support to this thesis. They first give credit to haptic perception as being the basis for lateral mental representation and ultimately visual representation. They go on to say that this perception is more of the tactile kinesthetic order rather than merely haptic as these perceptions are developing during the sensorimotor phase of development. Piaget and Inhelder offered a cognitive component for understanding object relations and the realization of the external object. They describe perceptual space, or libidinal object constancy, as essential in the ultimate formation of mental representation as well as spatial notions. However, space is one of a topological nature rather than Euclidean and therefore does not have a realistic sense of spatial relationships but rather a naïve one. Piaget and Inhelder further explain that much of the reason for this is that the child has not yet developed the cognition for order or continuity, and so the child's graphic representations are in terms of proximity of elements rather than actual representation. Referring to the art of three-and-a-half-year-old children that they gathered, they do note that there is an element of separation in these early pictorial images in that elements will be represented in a way that their forms can be distinguished from each other. If Piaget had put a pencil in the hand of babies, as he mused, he might have gotten renderings like the ones gathered during my research with Kestenberg and drawn similar conclusions to ours.

There is a general trend in development that evolves from the horizontal plane in which the baby is first held and fed, takes the world in, and begins communication, through the vertical plane, in which the baby takes hold of things and drops or releases them, into the sagittal plane in which the baby goes towards and away from objects. Eventually the space is neither "me" nor "not-you" but rather "not-me" and "not-you."

This depersonalization allows us to conceptualize space as a construct rather than an actual experience. The developing child reanimates space by populating it with connection to objects. What Winnicott called the intermediate space is referred to in movement terminology as near space, a small space between mother and child when mother holds the baby or leans towards it closely. The slightest movements bring them in touch with one another, thus the "me" and "not-me" meet. The connection is established through breathing which brings them closer through inhalation and further away in exhalation. What in movement theory is called intermediate space is the communicational space in which one can easily see the object's face. (Kestenberg & Sossin, 1979).

In the horizontal plane, the distance between the objects is well established, and it is bridged over by reaching in space and in art by way of horizontal connecting lines. In the vertical plane, it is easier to reach as far as one can reach into a space. Vertical lines bridge over the distance between the child and the adults who stand high above. Lastly in the sagittal plane, the developing child overreaches and changes their kinesphere by moving away from a stable stance and transferring their whole body into space, going somewhere as a whole instead of just reaching from a stable position. Using all three planes creates multidimensional movement which gives a sculpture quality to images of ourselves and objects.

How does one develop one's own image and that of objects in relation to space? Reaching into space and moving back creates flowing boundaries and a feeling of elasticity and plasticity of our body. We become successively tense and free in our movement and at the same time, we become smaller (shrinking) and bigger (growing) (Kestenberg, 1967). The feeling of tension and release, of inhibition and facilitation of movement combined with the change in one's body space, whereby one shrinks away from and grows into space, gives the baby the feeling of being separate but able to reach out and take in. The more separate the baby feels, the smaller and more rigid they feel. The more the baby reaches out, the bigger and freer the baby feels. The child populates the near space with transitional objects. As this child goes out to the intermediate space of communication, the separation is there, but there are continuous attempts to bridge over them through movement, as one may see in the child feeding the mother during self-feeding and through carrying sounds from one to another.

Simultaneously with the development of this distinction, there begins an appreciation of living versus inanimate, which does not have the elasticity and plasticity of living tissue. Inanimate objects become incorporated into the baby's body image when enveloped with their hands and mouths and make them their own by receiving them into their space. The baby's warmth and their own elasticity are lent to the inanimate object, and they become endowed with an animate quality. Inanimate objects become bridges between ourselves and living objects that we can mirror and attune to (Searles, 1960).

The developing child projects themselves onto the inanimate objects and transforms them into the intermediate objects that are bridges to the baby's first love object (Winnicott, 1953). The mother's hand gives the child intermediate objects; the child's hand receives it. Many of these objects are tools for maternal care and self-care. If they have qualities which remind the child of the qualities of the animate, either through their texture, their sound or smell, or some visual similarities, they can become transitional objects which are both "me" and "not-me." Because the baby can hold onto them and need not give them up except voluntarily, these inanimate objects help the baby to overcome the pain of losses during and after separation.

Object Relations and Developmental Theory Applications to Treatment

Margret Mahler's stages towards separation/individuation (Mahler, Pine, & Bergman, 1975) give us a clear way of understanding the path that early development takes within typical parameters. When understanding object relations, it is useful to look at the entire separation/individuation process. It is during this process that the child begins to play and practice with the separation from the primary object which is usually the mother. Of particular interest is the stage that Mahler calls *Rapprochement*. This usually appears between 15 and 18 months and continues until or through three years of life. This range on either end is dependent on the child's own personality as well as on external events in the child's life. The mother/child pair has developed a relationship to each other through resolution of previous stages that is now played out in this stage. Ideally, they were able to be attached optimally during the earlier stage of typical symbiosis so that the child now has internal awareness of the internal images and clear description of our ability to maintain symbols within our psyche.

Horner (1979) discusses the successful resolution of the rapprochement subphase as significant to later healthy development. She describes the lack of resolution in this phase as the basis for borderline and narcissistic personality disorders based on failures in integration and self-cohesion, a tendency towards fusion and away from autonomy and a tendency towards splitting good and bad objects.

Obernbreit (1985) discusses the value of the language of art and how artists learn methods of art as valuable tools and can additionally apply the language of art to address intrapsychic phenomenon. Art therapists can, therefore, "conceptually translate back and forth from an Object Relations framework to the 'language' of art" (p.18). For example, artists understand the importance of placement of objects in a composition for the balance of a piece. An art therapist may simply remark to the patient that the objects in the composition are close to or far from each other. This is not an interpretation as much as an observation brought to the patient's attention for insight into their object relations.

There are good reasons for creative arts therapists to be informed about object relations theory. Every person brings a personal history to a session. Understanding their development is crucial to doing effective therapy. An awareness of the path of human development within typical parameters must be understood to best understand patients and disruptions along their way and to facilitate the journey of the treatment. The patient before the therapist is the same person who was once a baby, a child, an adolescent, and brings this information to the session, which is part of the big picture. People will repeat patterns from their own development so disregarding their history will result in ineffective treatment.

Robbins (1989) applies the theory of object relations to the process and products of the creative arts therapies in *The Psychoaesthetic Experience: An Approach to Depth-oriented Treatment*. Through clinical examples, he demonstrates how the elements of self, object, and the interplay of these within the intermediate space of the therapeutic session allow the therapist insight into developmental issues and deficits that need to be addressed in treatment. What can often be masked or misunderstood in verbal messages may be able to be seen more clearly in graphic expression.

> …there are multiple levels of consciousness entering into the engagements, as the relationships from each person's past make contact, become enmeshed, and occasionally lose sight of one another.
>
> Art adds a dimension to this engagement. Sometimes the art mirrors or deepens what is going on in the relationship. In other instances, the

art form may offer something diametrically opposed to the verbal dialogue. This added dimension gives us a new perspective on our internal
relationships as it brings us to new levels of consciousness.

(Robbins in Rubin, 1987, p. 65)

The Significance of Early Scribbles

Objects have certain shapes and textures that hands and eyes can explore.
They become the child's own creation when they make them into their
own and share them with the mother, who offered them but did not animate them. Ability to animate the inanimate becomes the core of transitional
phenomena and of art. By defining the space that surrounds the self and
the object, the inanimate objects make space part of our living experience.
A drawing tool can be an object to explore and can be an animate tool to
reach a surface which becomes a concrete and symbolic substitute for the
three-dimensional space.

Goldhahn (2011) suggests that if we look at early art from an object-
relational perspective, the mark made on the paper represents a secure
encounter with objects. The child can now change, manipulate, and make
the object one's own. These scribbles are marks that communicate *a having
been there*, a relevant message both to the self and to others.

While all developmental art theorists recognize the importance of early
scribbles to the development of graphic representation and symbol formation, it is my research with my mentor, Dr. Judith Kestenberg, that offers
significance to these scribbles as indicators of the development of object
relations. This will be discussed extensively in the next chapter. There is
no doubt that the baby develops a sense of objects and remembers them
visually, acoustically, through movement and other ways. Winnicott's intermediate space (1971a) between "me" and "not-me" is where transitional
objects are dealt with. Most transitional objects are touched, carried,
brought close to the body, and dropped. We are reminded of the way the
young baby draws on paper, touching and dropping contact. Because the
transitional object can be found again and again, it has a permanent value
as a creation of one's own, picking it up and relinquishing it operates on
the same principles as the child's creating lines, stopping and recreating
them. Visual space created on canvas comes to life through the motion
of the brush, pen, or pencil on the medium. No picture could be created
without the artist's movements through space. As a matter of fact, the artist
could draw in the air which would create a dance that left no trace of the
movement on the surface.

Viktor Lowenfeld and W. L. Brittain (1957), describing early art
experiences as primarily kinesthetic in nature, remarked that if we put a
brush in a baby's mouth and recorded the movement, we would have baby
art. In drawings we see forms arising and lines crossing and crisscrossing
them as if communicating with the forms. Eventually, when these forms
are internalized and endowed with the images of one's body, space is again

used for communicating, showing, explaining, removing oneself, and coming back. The virtual space in art, the space of illusion, lends itself to symbolic representation of movement in space. It transforms the experience of the individual space into art or creative space. Such a transformation of practical, real, and actual space occurs without necessarily performing of visual art in Winnicott's intermediate space. Space is, by necessity, defined by boundaries, be they the horizon reached by the eye, or by four walls of a room. The limits of our vision and the limits imposed by the environment and by people create the condition in which we recognize that space exists. Without boundaries, we experience no space.

Schilder (1935) pointed out that the body image incorporates objects and spreads itself in space. Every movement goes into space and back to the body, the most basic motor rhythm. Going out into space, we encounter obstacles or boundaries when we reach an object and can no longer move. The space is now delineated by the degree of movement necessary to reach an object. By drawing the object to ourselves as the baby does, we diminish the distance between self and object

Bergman (1978) describes in some detail how the child masters distance between self and mother in the process of separation/individuation. By bringing the object to oneself, we incorporate it into our body image. By the incessant interplay between taking in and losing the object, we create the personal space which divides into near, intermediate, and reach space. Within this personal space, our movement creates designs in space using lines and loops, large and small amplitudes, smooth and sharp changes in direction (Kestenberg and Sossin, 1979). This design is translated into pictorial design on paper creating that multidimensional space.

Having created lines and spatial units on paper, we divide and encircle space and gain mastery over it, populating it by shapes enclosed by our own boundaries in addition to the boundary limitations imposed by the environment, in the case of drawing, by the size and form of the paper. Thus, going out into space creates shapes in space and boundaries between shapes. At least some of these shapes are projections of our own shape and of its position in space. As we go out into space, to the "not-me" area, we give something to this space that is not our own, and when we return to our own body, we take something from the "not-me" into the "me."

Early art representations seem to express the child's kinesthetic feelings about self. From going out tentatively into space and from being rhythmic about lines going away and coming back, the child develops a continuity of venturing into space as well as a feeling for a base near the floor and the erect body going into space above. With locomotion providing more distance to traverse, the drawings cover a larger area going from one side of the page diagonally upwards to the other side. The growing baby and toddler seem to reproduce feelings about themselves as a moving being. Moving into space allows for contact and the back and forth of contact and separation are represented in seemingly endless lines going towards each other crossing and crisscrossing. The paper space becomes a container for projecting one's

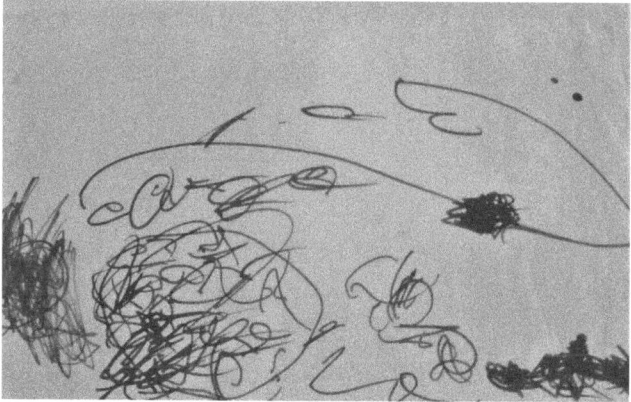

Figure 2.1 Giving form to space and shape

kinesthetic and postural image of the body and creating contact with other images. From the dynamic images of the first year, there emerges more stable, grounded images in the second year. In the third year, the newly established stability in which form has begun to be differentiated, there develops a new mobility in which space is not traversed every which way, but there is a definite movement from one side of the paper to the other. Not until the end of this year does a visual image evolve with rounded boundaries. Eventually the never-ending spiral becomes a circle, in which only one rather than many images remain. Movement quality ceases and a static shape is extrapolated from the forever changing rhythmic changes in shape. The child populates near space with transitional objects. As the child goes out to the intermediate space of communication, the separation is there, but there are continuous attempts to bridge over them through movement. In drawings, we see forms arising and lines crossing and crisscrossing them as if communicating with the forms. Eventually, when these forms are internalized and endowed with the images of one's body, space is again used for communicating, showing, explaining, removing oneself, and coming back.

3 The Kestenberg Art Profile

Dr. Judith Kestenberg's Contribution to Developmental Art Profile

It was both my personal and professional pleasure to work with Dr. Judith Kestenberg, internationally renowned child psychiatrist and psychoanalyst. I worked as the art therapist in her Center for Parents and Children sponsored by Child Development Research (CDR) for many years and then continued to do research with her after her Center closed and while I was running a Center of my own based on her model. CDR was a program where typically developing children engaged in play that incorporated art, movement, and music, and all children were accompanied by a parent. Not only was I the art therapist at the Center, but I was a mother there with three of my four children. Dr. Kestenberg's knowledge of infant and child development was encyclopedic and working with her and watching her with the children was an education for me in this area, which could not be matched by any other clinical experiences I have had. I learned a great deal as well from her assistant, Arnhilt Buelte and the dance/movement therapist, Susan Loman. Arnhilt Built was involved in developing the Kestenberg Movement Profile along with Dr. Kestenberg and the Sands Point Movement Study Group. Susan Loman and K. Mark Sossin conducted research and furthered the clinical application of the Kestenberg Movement Profile (KMP). The KMP is a system of movement notation related to infant movements and is studied internationally by dance/movement therapists, psychotherapists, and movement researchers. Loman and Sossin along with Janet Kestenberg Amighi co-authored the 2018 textbook outlining the KMP and its applications, *The Meaning of Movement: Embodied Developmental, Clinical, and Cultural Perspectives of the Kestenberg Movement Profile, Volume II*. Susan Loman and Rose Brandt (1992) edited *The Body-Mind Connection in Human Movement Analysis*, which is a volume including much of the research we did at CDR and chapters that clarify and elucidate many of the clinical aspects of the KMP.

A personal reason for wanting to write this book is to write down some of the stories of my work with Judith Kestenberg. I consider it a privilege to have worked and done research with Dr. Kestenberg for ten years. It is becoming a professional mission of mine to write down the stories of some of my mentors who influenced generations of creative arts therapists and I am encouraging others to do the same about their influential mentors. This oral history, if you will, will preserve personal snapshots of how these icons of our profession taught and supervised those of us who had the honor of knowing and learning from them. This personal knowledge about them, in turn, enhances their theories and makes them more understandable.

Dr. Kestenberg came to the USA in 1937, losing her parents in the Holocaust. Hearing from child survivors how different their experiences were, she helped established foundations and programs devoted to child survivors and children of survivors. Her husband helped survivors receive reparations from the Germans and interviewed child survivors around the world. They trained others in special psychological-oriented interviewing techniques. The 1,500 interviews are archived at Hebrew University in Israel.

Dr. Kestenberg was a character. Her spirit was indomitable, her energy endless, and her knowledge infinite. She was always right. One day, I watched her patiently listen to one of the fathers, who was also a psychiatrist, as he elaborated on a theory he had, differing from Dr. Kestenberg's, regarding the reason for his child's behavior during a developmental stage. When he was finished, Dr. Kestenberg looked at him with a stern face and said, "Dr. R, you may think you are right, but I know I am right." And she was. In fact, she was the supervisor of psychiatric residents for many of the psychiatrists with whom I crossed paths over the years in my professional career—and most of them were afraid of her.

Although she was fairly deaf and clearly tone deaf, Dr. Kestenberg took singing lessons in her 80s, from one of the CDR Moms, who was a music therapist, because she wanted to be able to sing with the children. In fact, when she and her husband were involved with interviewing Holocaust survivors from the former Soviet Union, they both studied Russian, again in their 80s, to be able to speak to these people in their own language.

Creative arts therapists think of Winnicott's transitional space as the magical place between infant and mother in which creativity and imagination are born. One day during staff supervision, Dr. Kestenberg told a story of someone asking Winnicott the question: What exactly is transitional space? Dr. Kestenberg said that he crooked his arm with the palm open towards his face and said, "About this far," and she mimicked the motion that Winnicott had made. One could imagine a baby in the crook of a loving arm gazing into the *object's* eyes creating a wonderful, and very essential, connection from which the relationship and creativity grow and flourish.

The work and writings of Dr. Kestenberg contribute significantly to creative arts therapy theory related to human development and sexuality, object relations and object loss, and parenting. Dr. Kestenberg's work is groundbreaking regarding the body rhythms of typically developing infants and the effects of the interaction with the *object* and the *holding environment*. Her research explores the development of creativity, which is invaluable in the study of creative arts therapy. Awareness of Dr. Kestenberg's research sheds light on developmental issues of patients of all ages and can inform best practice.

However, my primary reason for writing this book is to finally and officially publish the Kestenberg Art Profile, which evolved over many years of the research that Dr. Kestenberg and I did at the CDR in Sands Point, New York. This center was exactly as it says it was. We studied and did research with typically developing children, ages birth through three, who attended CDR with a parent. Most of the parents were professionals, and some engaged in research with Dr. Kestenberg, and others offered presentations on their professional work specific to child development. Because I strongly believe that understanding developmental art can support an art therapist's knowledge base and best practice, when I taught graduate students, I taught developmental art courses. And I taught the KAP to graduate art therapy students for years, but it has never been officially published. Two CDR art therapy interns contributed significantly to parts of our research—Erika Leeuwenburg and Sharon Burns. Both have gone on to many years of respectable art therapy practice.

Origins of the KAP

The KAP very much grew out of the Kestenberg Movement Profile (KMP). The KMP is a standardized system of movement notation used by dance/movement therapists internationally. Through notating and graphing an individual's body movement, dance/movement therapists interpret the results and determine a psychological profile. The KMP reflects two lines of development. System I focuses on the tension flow-effort line of development describing movement dynamics, and System II focuses on the shape flow, shaping on the developmental line and describes relational development and the structure of movements (Hastie, 2006).

The KMP was developed by Dr. Kestenberg's Sands Point Movement Study Group (Kestenberg, 1967). Kestenberg describes the influence of Freud in the evolution of the KMP through his theorizations about instinctual drives and instinctual energy—oral, anal, and phallic. He based these theories on both neurophysiological models and actual direct observations of movements, specifically observing the tension and relaxation of muscles during certain affective and ideational states. The KMP includes stages along the psychosexual continuum not in Freud's original construct. Anna Freud (1963) offered the significance of the urethral stage in the developmental line. She pointed to the function of the urethra as the area of libidinal cathexis during this time of development, therefore offering a distinct period of id and ego interaction in the development of personality.

> Since the desired aim on this line is not the comparatively intact survival of drive derivatives but the control, modification, and transformation of the urethral and anal trends, the conflicts between id, ego, superego, and environmental forces become particularly obvious.
>
> (p. 253)

Kestenberg (1968) introduced the inner genital phase as a distinct period of ruminations and fantasies of being pregnant and is relevant for boys and girls. And Kestenberg (1968) renamed the phallic phase as the outer genital, again allowing the physical, exploring, curious, and outward energy of this phase for boys and girls.

"Periodic alterations in muscle tension create discernible patterns called **tension flow rhythms**" (Kestenberg Amighi, Loman, Lewis, & Sossin, 1999, p. 24). An observer of these rhythms notates them utilizing the standardized tension flow writing system. The Sands Point Movement Study Group observed that particular tension flow rhythms were emanating from specific biological zones and reflected related biological functions. For example, the sucking rhythm of the mouth is necessary for breastfeeding, and the squeeze/release rhythm of the anal sphincter allows for defecation. Patterned changes in muscle tension are alterations between free and bound flow—between the agonist and antagonist muscles. The pleasant release of energy by the agonist muscles is free flow; the inhibiting constraint of the antagonist muscles is bound flow (Kestenberg & Sossin, 1979).

The tension flow rhythms each have two phases—the indulgent and the fighting. The indulgent phase is the beginning of each developmental stage, and the fighting phase completes the stage. In this naming of fighting, the meaning has to do with the pursuit of mastery in the phase and not aggression in the way that we typically understand it. The terms aggressive and sadistic are used interchangeably with fighting, even throughout this text. The child modifies through these drives. The indulgent phase begins the stage following mastery from the previous stage. The baby practices and incorporates new material, and it culminates with mastery in the fighting phase. The chart below is reprinted with permission from Taylor & Francis and is from *The Meaning of Movement: Developmental and Clinical Perspectives of the Kestenberg Movement Profile* (Kestenberg Amighi, Loman, Lewis, & Sossin, 1999, **Table 1** Tension Flow Rhythms, p. 27).

The next component of the KMP is tension flow attributes. "Tension flow rhythms arise in response to physiological as well as biological needs… personality and emotions shape the way needs are met" (Kestenberg Amighi, Loman, Lewis, & Sossin, 1999, p. 59). We exhibit different qualities

Table 3.1 Tension flow rhythms

Tension Flow Rhythms		
Oral	Sucking	Snapping/Biting
Anal	Twisting	Strain/Release
Urethral	Running/Drifting	Starting/Stopping
Inner Genital	Swaying	Surging/Birthing
Outer Genital	Jumping	Spurting/Ramming

Table 3.2 In KAP: Art driven by rhythms

Phase	Indulgent rhythm	Fighting rhythm
Oral	Light lines	Stabbing/Dotting
Anal	Lines get denser, moving across the page	Lines become more upright
Urethral	Lines flow; more page is filled	Zigzag lines/"my name"
Inner genital	Lines begin to form circles	Circles differentiate/ connectors
Outer genital (less rhythm driven and more personality driven)	Forms have distinct shapes	Stories emerge in the art/ Fascination with human figure

of tension flow, called *attributes,* in our behavior and even experience different qualities of tension flow in our bodies. For example, someone may hold something with bound flow; someone else with neutral of free flow. The attributes of flow as they move from free through neutral to bound are: flow adjustment to even flow; low intensity to high intensity; and gradual to abruptness. "Tension flow attributes introduce a measure of control or regulation over the expression of needs (rhythms) through the influence of feelings and temperament" (Kestenberg Amighi, Loman, Lewis, & Sossin, 1999, p. 73).

When considering visual arts, tension flow attributes can be translated to observe the way someone approaches art materials, surfaces, and execution. One young artist may approach the art activity abruptly, hold on tight to the marker and get right to work—even flow and high intensity. Another young artist may gradually approach the task, may sort through the markers, and get to work thoughtfully—flow adjustment and low intensity.

The next components of the KMP are *pre-efforts* and *efforts.* Rudolph Laban (1966) contributed to the knowledge base of Dance/Movement Therapy with a system of movement notation he developed through his observation of dancers responding to the environmental forces of space, weight, and time. Laban identified these movement qualities as *efforts.* In relation to space, one can be direct or indirect; in relation to weight, one can exhibit strength or lightness; in relation to time, one accelerates or decelerates.

Through observing infants and toddlers, Kestenberg and Sossin (1979) concluded that these efforts were not yet fully developed, so they identified the related precursors of these efforts as *pre-efforts.* The quality of each pre-effort resembles the effort in its less mature, less regulated form and reflects the baby's work towards refinement and mastery of each effort.

The chart below is a compilation of *Table 3* The Developmental Line System 1. (p. 77) and *Table 4* The Developmental Line from Pre-Efforts to Efforts. (p. 91) and reprinted with permission from Taylor & Francis and is from *The Meaning of Movement: Developmental and Clinical Perspectives*

Table 3.3 Tension flow attributes: pre-efforts and efforts

Tension flow attributes	Pre-efforts	Efforts
	Approaching **space** with	
Even flow	Channeling	Direct
Flow adjustment	Flexibility	Indirect
	Approaching **weight** with	
High intensity	Vehemence/Straining	Strength
Low intensity	Gentleness	Lightness
	Approaching **time** with	
Abruptness	Suddenness	Acceleration
Graduality	Hesitation	Deceleration

of the Kestenberg Movement Profile (Kestenberg Amighi, Loman, Lewis, & Sossin, 1999).

Envision and compare a baby's effort in a task to an adult's to better understand the pre-efforts to efforts continuum. Consider the task of reaching for an object that fell off of and went under a table. An adult would reach for it directly and use some indirect effort to reach behind the table leg where it fell. The adult's effort to pick the object up would reflect knowledge of weight. How quickly the adult approached the task would most likely be determined by knowledge of urgency. As the baby is still developing a relationship with space, weight, and time, and may not have previous knowledge of the object, their approach would follow all the steps as the adult's but with pre-efforts.

Another component of the KMP is *shape flow*. As the baby moves through space with pre-efforts, dimensionality happens. "Shape flow gives structure or form to tension flow by providing specific spatial components with which the dynamic qualities conform" (Kestenberg Amighi, Loman, Lewis, & Sossin, 1999, p. 110). Bipolar shape flow reflects growing and shrinking; unipolar shape flow reflects attraction and repulsion. For the infant, this begins on the horizontal dimension-side to side, then for an upright toddler on the vertical dimension, up and down; and finally, for the burgeoning child, on the sagittal dimension, forward and backward. Imagine time elapse photography to get a sense of how one understands shape flow.

As an artist and art therapist observing and notating on infants and toddlers at CDR, I started to see how strongly connected movements were to their art products. Developmental movement elements translated to the infants' and toddlers' art expression. Artists task themselves with making shapes and approaching space, weight, and time with an effort to create something where there was not something. Dance and visual art seemed to be relatives as we observed and notated the infants and toddlers, and we began collecting data and presenting on rudimentary aspects (Loman & Brandt, 1992). Dr. Kestenberg pointed out to me that the baby's art moved along the page as they began to crawl. I noticed their lines were more vertical when they began to stand. She pointed out that the babies made vehement stabbing motions while they were teething, and I began to see these dots as having to do with separation issues, even in the art of older children and adults. We discussed that teething is a portal for separation. Many mothers start the weaning process as the baby grows teeth and may bite. I observed that lines turned into forms as the child was becoming more sagittal, and then into separate forms, which I thought were people, most likely baby and mom. Dr. Kestenberg observed that there was a connector line between these figures that seemed to come and go during the separation/individu- ation process (Mahler, 1968). She also pointed out zigzag lines, which appear during the fighting subphase of the urethral phase. Dr. Kestenberg often asked the children what it was, and they replied it was their signed name. She also asked them what was going on in the picture, and we began to see whole stories in the children's art. We moved our research into three-dimensional art, different art media, use of photo images, and some exploration of the vertical plane for artmaking. For a reason I cannot explain, children draw at a higher level of development when working in the vertical plane than in the horizontal. For example, clear representations of human forms may appear in a child's art if working on an easel or blackboard but not so when working on a table.

And so, the KAP was born out of the KMP and observations and notations of the children as they danced and moved, made art, made music, and engaged in play. I will elaborate further. I have mentioned several times that I did KMP notation for our research. I wrote notations for the children at CDR and for my own children. I notated my own babies' movements in my womb and wrote down my dreams for research that Dr. Kestenberg was doing cor- relating the fetal rhythms to the dream content. But, alas, even though I did all the coursework for the KMP, I never finished my final assignment because life got in the way, and I was never officially certified. However, I use the KMP all the time in my work and understand its implications for practice.

Components of the KAP

In the KAP, linear, two-dimensional art aligns with the psychosexual phases of development and the KMP associated rhythms, both indulgent and fighting already discussed (see Table 3.2.): oral, anal, urethral, inner genital, outer genital. And the pre-efforts related to space, weight, and time can be understood in the KAP through observing the child's actual approach to and engagement in the artmaking process. Shape flow design, defined in the KMP, can be applied to the understanding of the space on a two-dimensional surface and to the development of three-dimensional art. Looking at the KAP from the developmental perspective:

- Development of line: oral, anal, urethral
- Development of form: urethral, inner genital
- Development of shape: outer genital

Psychosexual theory defines these as oral being the first year of life (0–1), anal being the second (1–2), urethral being the third (2–3), inner genital being the fourth (3–4), and outer genital being the fifth (4–5). My professional observation would place these stages accordingly: oral, 0–10 months; anal, 10–20 months; urethral, 20–30 months; inner genital 30–48 months; outer genital, starting at 48 months. Of course, there is overlap within and between each stage.

When studying human development, there is a tendency to think of it as linear—chronological. But typical child development is three steps forward and one back. This is healthy regression for the purpose of gaining mastery over a stage. Human beings jump forward to test the waters but happily return to the shore to regroup and move forward again. That is how we learn and grow. Kestenberg (1968) states that the assigned boundaries of the developmental phases are not always so distinct as there is overlapping in the progression related to constitutional or environmental influences. Precursors of phase-specific traits can be seen before they become dominant in a phase.

The presentation of human developmental theory is always linear. Theory reflects the norm, and everyone achieves developmental milestones around the same time and place but a little differently from each other. By working from this paradigm, we can better understand typical human development, and, therefore, be able to identify what is atypical. Most babies are walking by around one year of age. Some start earlier and some later. But typical human developmental theory gives us a window. Pediatricians, for example, may be concerned if a baby does not walk within that window and direct parents to seek a physical therapy evaluation. This is good. Similarly, as an art therapist, when I observe artwork made by a child, adolescent, or adult, I consider their chronological age compared to the product. This can give me a window into an event or issues occurring during a particular stage of development. For example, if a six-year-old child is not drawing human figures but does draw forms on the page, I would explore what was happening in their life during the time that forms were emerging to better understand why human figures have not yet appeared in their art.

Oral

The oral phase correlates with 0–10 months of age. The development of line in graphic art begins during the oral phase. The indulgent rhythm of the oral phase is sucking. That is the baby's job—to suckle. Dr. Kestenberg used to say that babies think and learn by tasting the world. In the KMP notation, this rhythm pervades the baby's body.

During our research, the mother seats herself with the baby on her lap at the table covered with paper, and she helps the child to bring the pencil to the paper by leaning forward or bringing the child's hand closer to the paper. The mother now holds the child's hand without restraining or guiding it, holding the hand without influencing movement. There are two reasons for guiding the baby's hand. One is that the child may easily drop the pencil, and the other is that the child may hold the pencil in such a way that it moves sideways with the fisted hand parallel to the paper. Paintbrushes or markers may still make a mark on the paper if held sideways, but, by virtue of their construction, pencils do not leave a trace if used sideways. With pencils, the mother must help the child hold the fisted hand as vertically as possible to the paper. When making contact with the drawing implements to the paper, the baby makes light strokes representing this sucking rhythm and gentle pre-effort. Because the baby moves in a horizontal plane during the oral phase, the lines are on the horizontal plane. The result are short, shaky lines, then longer and usually scattered in a lower corner of the paper. Since our original research, I have had more success using markers and then need to hold the baby's hand less.

The location of the lines on paper gradually shifts from one lower corner to the middle of the paper, depending on which hand the child uses. Sometimes the child holds two pencils, one in each hand, in which case the two middle sides of the paper are covered with lines.

Often, the infant is not looking at the page while drawing. Red is the preferential color of the infant (Bornstein, 1975), and there is much psycho-analytic literature devoted to the infant's attraction to the face while nursing and further identifying the face as the locus of personality development (Eigen, 1980). Therefore, to draw the baby's attention to the paper, we would often draw a red smiley face on the page. Our results were successful as the infants then began to draw lines with more intention, looking, touching, scratching, or stroking the paper.

The fighting rhythms of the oral phase are biting and snapping. As the baby moves towards food and self-feeding, biting and snapping are necessary rhythms for successful eating. Self-feeding is the first true separation from the mother because the baby is no longer helpless and needing only the breast. Babies are often teething during these months, so biting and snapping become part of their repertoire. The teething baby often makes jabbing, often jerking, motions when reaching for things, which has a similar energy

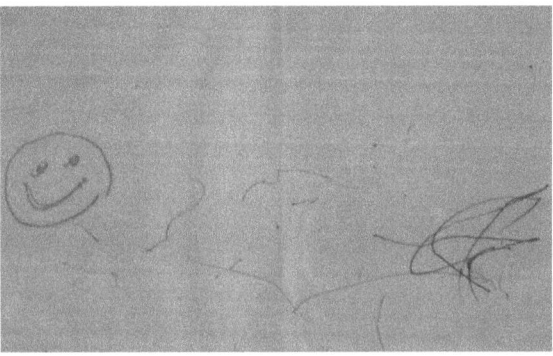

Figure 3.1 Red face drawn by adult to engage baby's eye contact

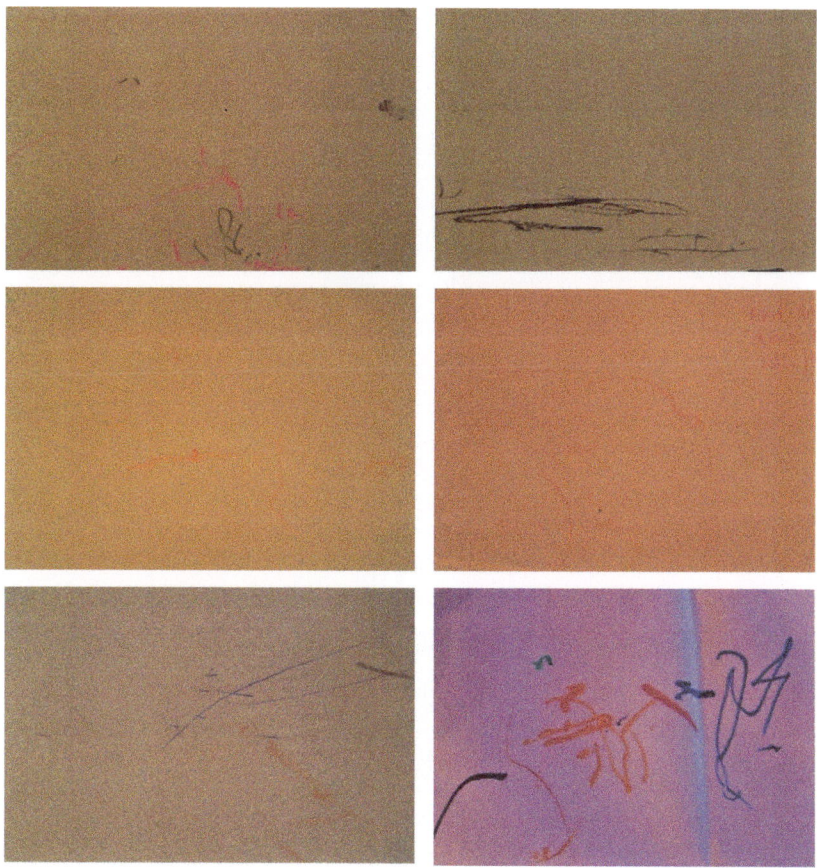

Chart 3.1a Oral indulgent lines/ Shaky light lines

to snapping and biting. While the short strokes are reminiscent in their rhythmic repetitions of sucking rhythms, the sharp strokes are reminiscent of the biting and snapping rhythms which teething brings into prominence.

In linear development, these rhythms translate to lines that are stabbing and dotting, and they are usually executed with vehemence. Whenever we noticed these lines, we would ask the mother if the baby were teething, and the answer was invariably yes. We concluded that these lines were an expression of this first separation, particularly when observing the vehemence that could have been expressing both physical and psychological pain. I have observed these oral dottings in the artwork of older children and adults dealing with separation issues. I have seen children whose families were dealing with divorce and custody battles draw dots on the page and then connect them like a dot-to-dot game. My sense is that they are trying to bring their family back together.

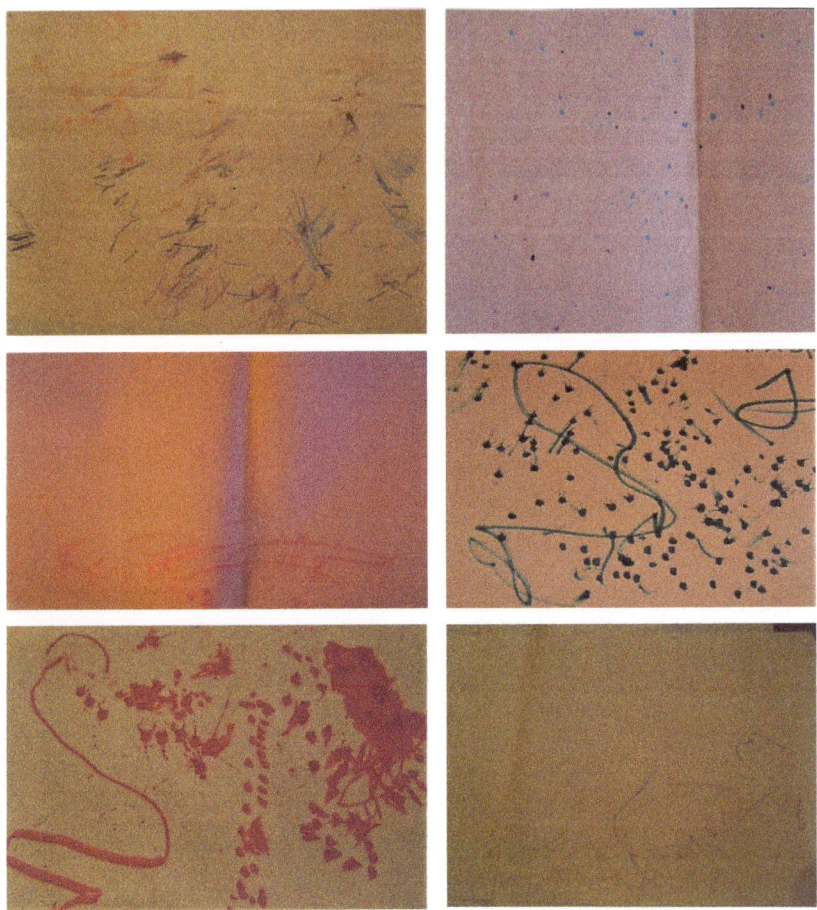

Chart 3.1b Oral fighting/Stabbing, dotting

Anal

The anal phase correlates to 10–20 months of age. As babies move through the oral phase and into the anal phase, they become more physically adept. Fewer objects go into the mouth and are, rather, examined through a clutching touch and visually. They creep and crawl and explore their environment. During the anal indulgent phase, this movement can be seen in the art in that they begin to draw lines that move across the page. By the time the baby begins to pull up from the floor, the horizontal lines get longer and venture from one side of the paper to the other. These lines are often repeated and crossed over. At first, they look like a delicate network, but as the baby experiences more anal rhythms, the lines become denser and cover much of the middle of the page. One gets the impression that the child

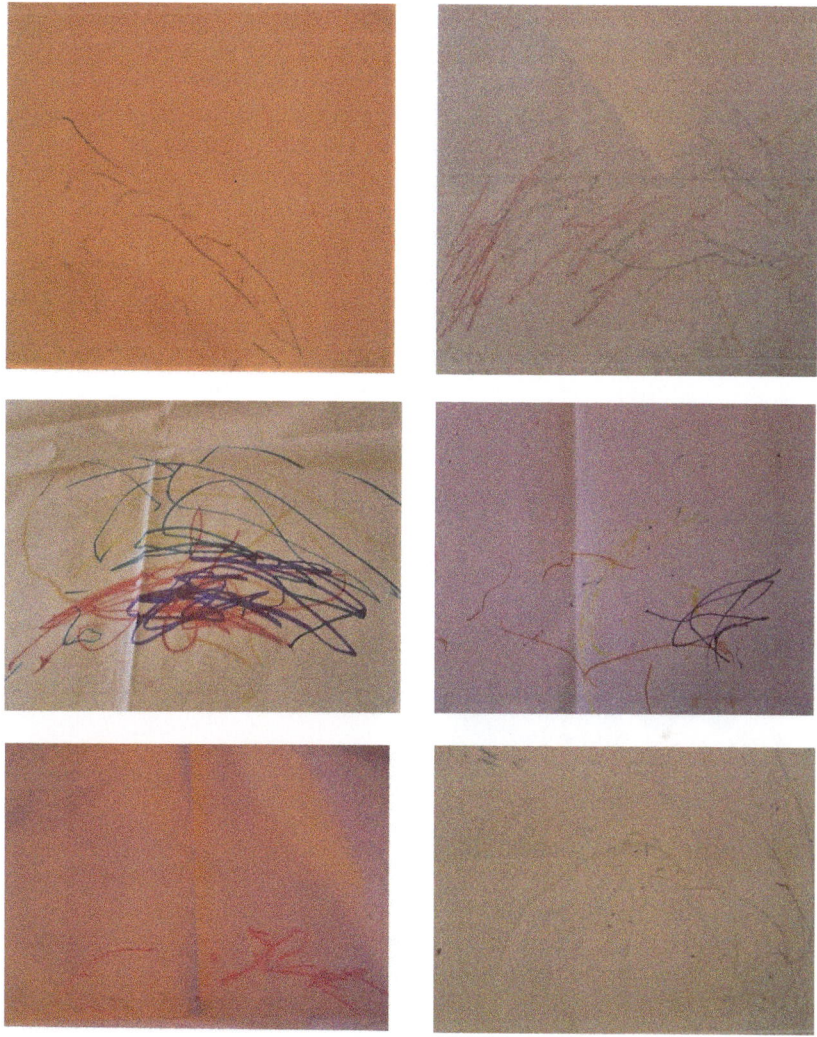

Chart 3.2a Anal indulgent/Creeping, crawling lines

experiences the chest as composed of a network of crisscrossing lines, while the continuity of chest and abdomen or pelvis are projected into longer lines with space surrounding created through lines in a harmonious way.

During the anal phase, the baby is now sitting and standing with mastery, moving well from horizontal to sitting to creeping and crawling to pulling oneself up to a vertical stand. The anal indulgent rhythm is twisting. This allows for a continual shift in perspective and of one's own weight and strength. Babies become more aware of the outside world but are still very connected to what is going on in their bodies. The area of cathexis is the anus and its job of elimination. They become more aware of and more interested in their bowel movements. Bowel movements are denser because the child is eating solid food, and it requires more effort to eliminate. The anal indulgent rhythm is straining. The baby's art reflects this during the anal indulgent phase in that it is denser and often created with vehemence. The dense lines move towards and cover the middle of the page with space remaining below, above, and on both sides. The picture is centered while the baby's torso appears to be centered and solid looking. There are some rudimentary forms caused by going back and forth.

Babies leaving the oral phase behind and moving into the anal phase are quickly becoming vertical creatures. The world is expanding even more as they stand up and look around. They are vertical but still two-dimensional.

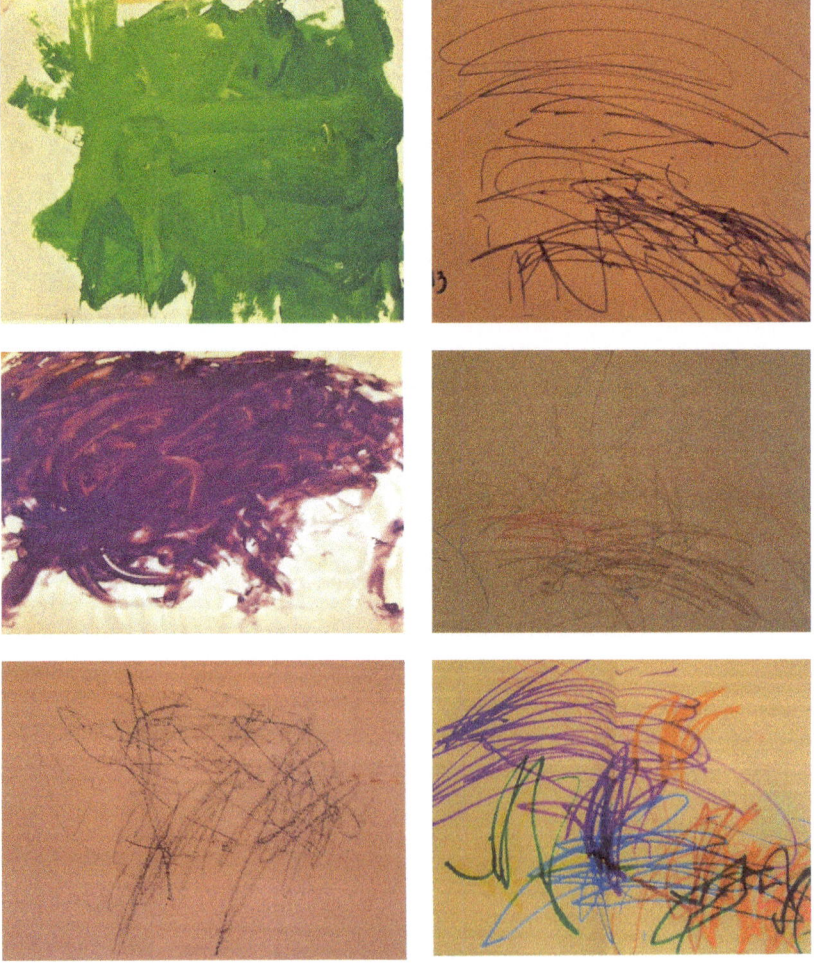

Chart 3.2b Anal indulgent/Dense lines

They do not yet have the integration of left–right movement. The best way to describe it is the *Gumby*® phase. Gumby is a Claymation character who appears to be flat in the vertical plane. Observe a child beginning to walk, and this makes sense. As artists, they are still two-dimensional, if you will, because they make lines and not forms, but as they move through the anal phase and master their ability to be upright, the lines begin to reflect their ascension to verticality—anal fighting. The vertical lines may reach the upper part of the paper. The lines may reverse and cross each other, closing off space, but they

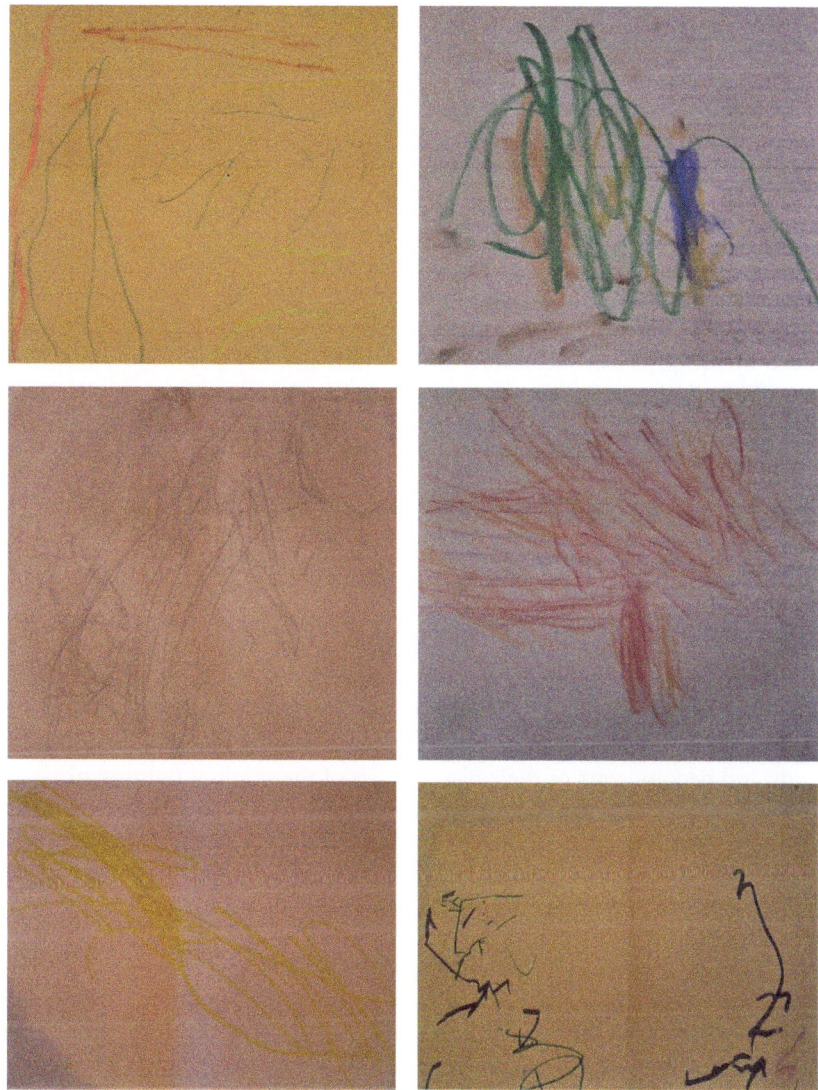

Chart 3.2c Anal fighting/Vertical lines

are not yet circles. Sometimes, the child will draw a dense base with vertical lines ascending from this, as if giving themselves something to stand on.

Urethral

This phase was delineated by Anna Freud (1963) as distinct from the anal phase. This phase describes the child from approximately 20–30 months of age. In Western society, children are generally trained for urine and bowel movements at the same time, and it usually involves climbing onto a toilet. However, in societies where people squat to eliminate, bowel training happens first. This is much more logical in terms of muscle development. Larger muscle groups, like those needed for elimination, develop strength earlier than fine muscle groups, like those needed for urination. During the urethral phase, I would notice that my babies would often be dry in the morning when they woke up. This indicated to me that their urethral muscles were ready to use a toilet, so, therefore, their anal muscles were ready.

During this time, the child is vertical and quickly progresses from walking to running. Dr. Kestenberg described this running as related to the urethral rhythm of flowing urine. This running and drifting are the urethral indulgent rhythms. Similarly, their art becomes more expansive on the page, filling more of the page and becoming more open and less dense than the anal lines. Towards the end of the urethral phase, these lines begin to turn back on themselves creating rudimentary leaf-like forms. The moving child is also a verbal child and might state that the expansive lines running across that page are waves in the ocean or a car driving across the page. Water-related imagery is common, like a fish.

The urethral child is a running child. Part of their play may be a delight in stopping themselves by running into people or furniture—both of which can cause harm to all parties involved. As children move through the urethral phase, they become more adept at being vertical/sagitta land more forwardly/backwardly coordinated in their movements. Now, they can practice how to both start and stop. Again, Dr. Kestenberg relates this to urine flow. As children master starting and stopping the urine flow, these rhythms fill their body and become part of their play. The art of the urethral fighting phase is strikingly connected to this as children begin to make zigzag lines—starting, stopping, changing direction. As already mentioned, children towards the end of the phase will tell us that it is their name or their signature. And when observing them doing this, it seems apparent that they are imitating the way that adults write.

Another component of the starting and stopping of urethral flow is controlling the flow. Once the child realizes that the flow does not have to end and restart abruptly, they regulate the flow. The child no longer crashes into things to stop, but rather begins to stop themselves, even making a turn and running back. At the point when children are doing this physically, they are doing it in their art.

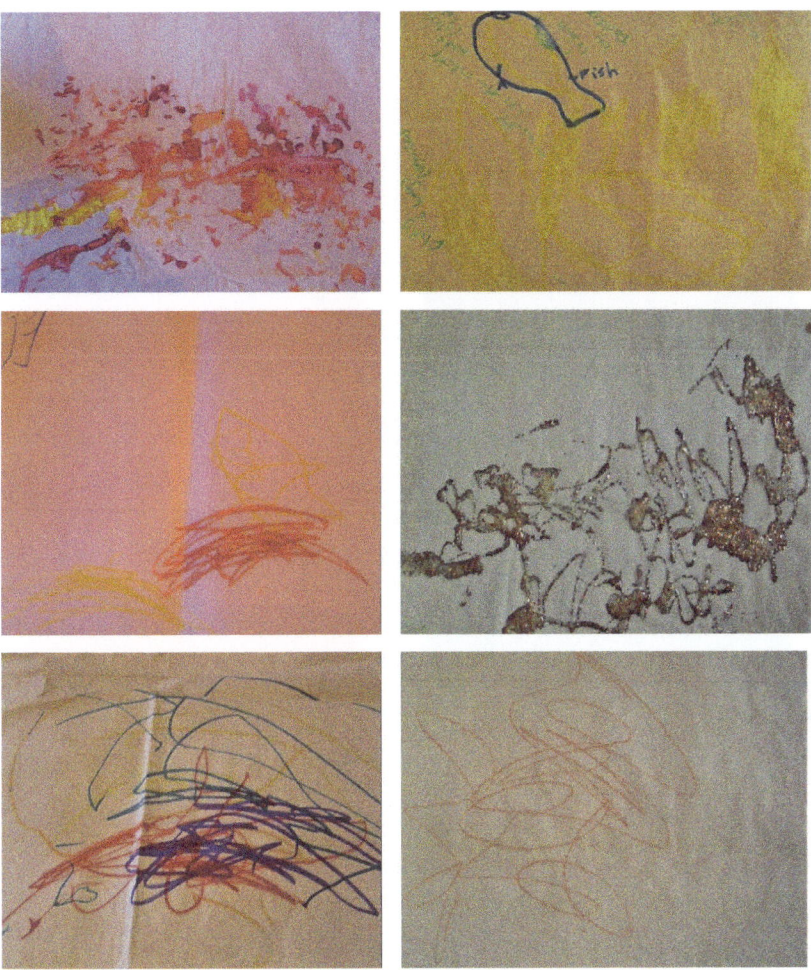

Chart 3.3a Urethral indulgent/Expanding lines/Looping back

Inner Genital

The inner genital phase was a contribution by Dr. Kestenberg (1968) to the developmental line continuum. She felt the need to recognize the specific developmental lines of femininity and revise the traditional developmental hierarchy of libidinal phases, acknowledging that both sexes progress through a feminine and phallic stage.

The inner genital phase follows the urethral phase and precedes the outer genital phase and correlates with the ages two-and-a-half to four years, or 30–48 months of age. During this time, children, both boys and girls, become interested in where babies come from and often believe that they have babies growing inside of them because they see babies growing inside of mothers

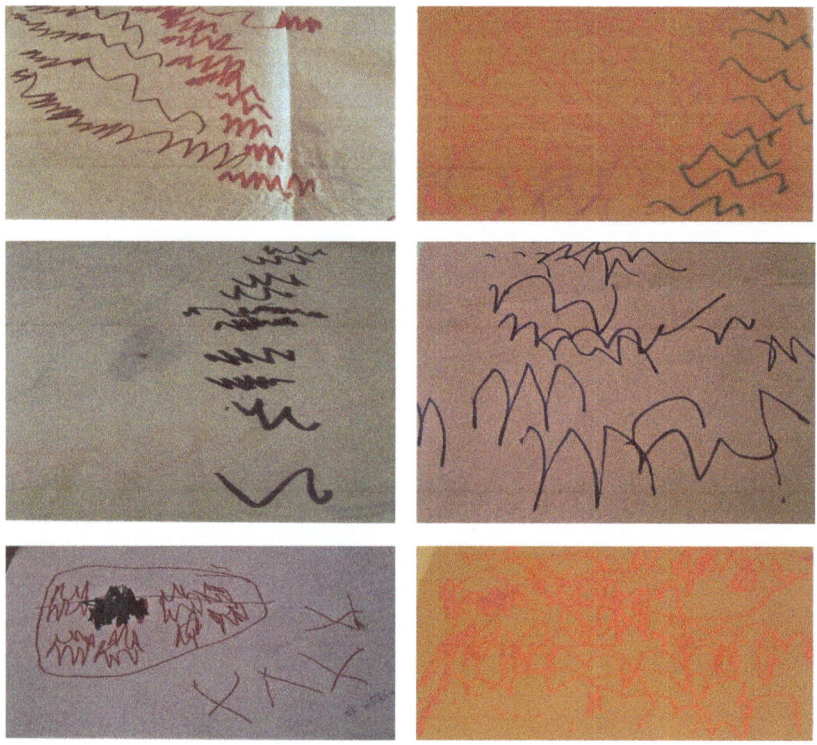

Chart 3.3b Urethral fighting/Zigzags

around them. The previously running child becomes pensive and philosoph-ical and asks many questions.

A characteristic of the inner genital child is an insistence on wearing certain outfits. Dr. Kestenberg believed that girls wanted to wear dresses because they had the illusion of wearing maternity clothing. This may be so, but many boys insist on wearing the same shirt each day. My older son wore a Superman outfit every day for months. Perhaps wearing the same outfit is deeply and unconsciously imbedded in believing your body is growing something inside, and the sameness protects that sense. But it may also have to do with wanting to control the world around by taking charge of yourself and making your own decisions. All these hypotheses relate to birthing one's self in the individuation process—the biggest work of this phase.

Dr. Kestenberg very much believed that children were not ready for sep-aration from their parents until age four. She called ages three to four, the *second chance*. Dr. Kestenberg felt that the three-year-old child has verbal skills and, can therefore, clarify and resolve preverbal experiences. Dr. Kestenberg felt this stage was essential for the child's developing ego and to support sep-aration/individuation and further growth.

During this phase of development, the child has incorporated horizontal and vertical and has progressed to the sagittal plane. Their sense of direction and shape is now three-dimensional. Their art representations follow this pattern. During the end of the urethral fighting phase and blending with the inner genital indulgent phase, form appears. The ever-expanding lines of the urethral fighting phase come back on themselves and begin to form circles or the first form. Circles appear universally in children's art (Kellogg, 1967). At this age, children draw many lines going in every direction and combining with each other in a design. The paper space seems populated by shapes connecting, separating, and merging through crisscrossing. Separate forms become clear. They are identified as people or animals, and there is a sense that they are communicating with each other. During this phase, children will distinctly draw circular forms contained within other circular forms, often stating that these are babies growing inside mommies.

When children are in the inner genital fighting phase, they are more social beings. They have become more aware that they are separate from their parents and from each other and have a solid sense of me-not me. As

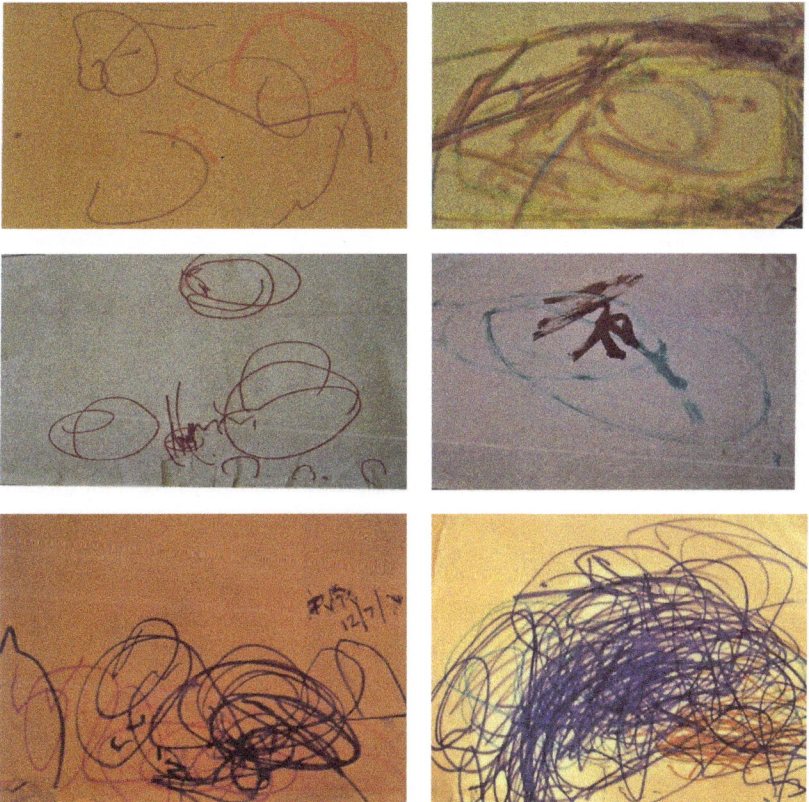

Chart 3.4a Inner genital indulgent/Circular and containing forms appear

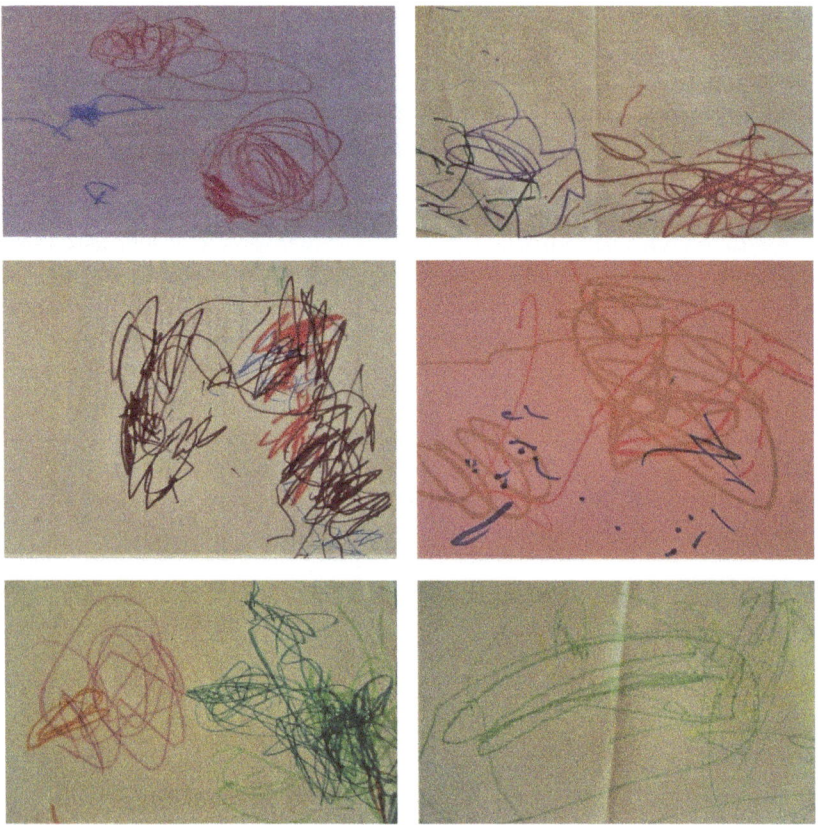

Chart 3.4b Inner genital fighting/Connectors come and go

already mentioned, during this phase children draw circles that are distinct and some that overlap or are contiguous to each other. The circles that are distinct sometimes have connector lines, and sometimes they do not. The separation and connection dynamic going on in the child's development is graphically represented.

Outer Genital

Kestenberg (1968) renamed Freud's phallic phase as the outer genital phase. The KMP rhythms observed during this phase are jumping (indulgent) and ramming/spurting (fighting). Her observations were that both boys and girls present with these rhythms. Just as boys become pensive and ruminative and have fantasies of having babies growing inside of them during the inner genital phase, girls are running, jumping, ramming, and spurting during the outer genital phase. In fact, the outer genital phase arrives on time for almost every child at exactly four years old, or 48 months. Children passing through this phase love to move around a great deal, and this is essential to their physical, emotional, behavioral, and cognitive development. They are taking in the world around them kinesthetically, with curiosity and energy.

At the risk of sounding gender incorrect, I will own my personal observations that boys in the outer genital stage love to play with cars, trucks, trains, tractors, and other vehicles. Girls in the outer genital stage seem to become more social with each other and seem to be more aware of and sensitive to social constructs like living with a family, weddings, and jobs. Boys were offered dolls and house toys, but they did not prefer to play with them. Girls were offered vehicles for free play, but they did not prefer to play with them, except for firetrucks, which are iconic toys for all four-year-old children. Dress-up is also a creative play activity enjoyed by all children of this age group.

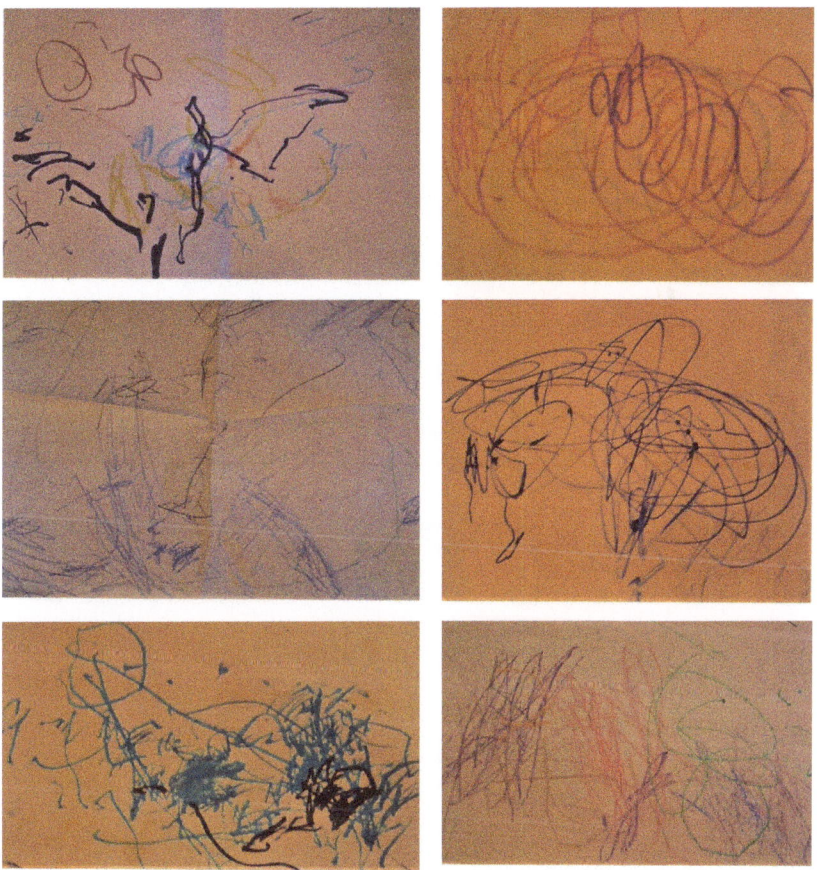

Chart 3.5a Outer genital indulgent/Shapes appear

One day at CDR, three soon-turning-four-year-old girls decided to dress as brides—one of the girls had recently been in her aunt's wedding party. They decided they needed a groom, so one of the girls approached a four-year-old boy who was engrossed in playing with a fleet of vehicles. She told him they were getting married and needed a groom. She insisted that he had to marry them. When she was ignored, she stormed away stating

Picking apples

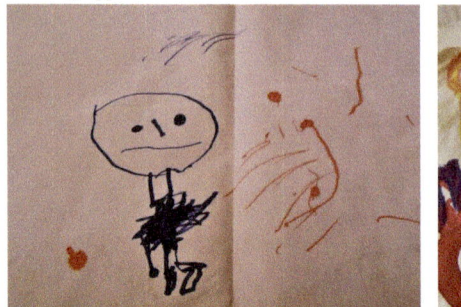
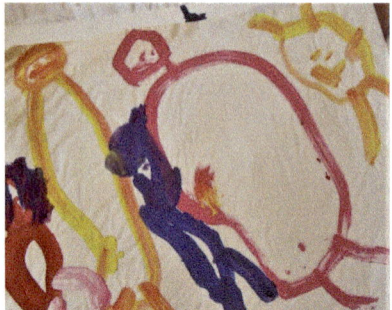

Taking the train to Rome

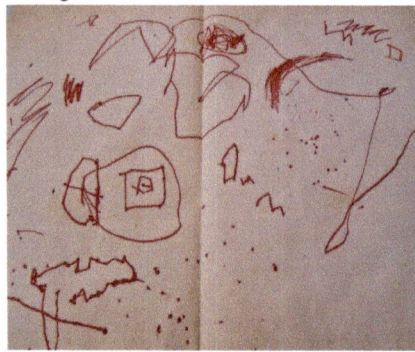
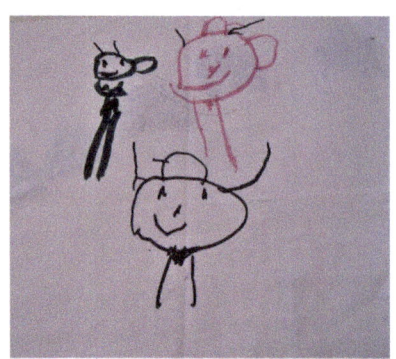

Teepee

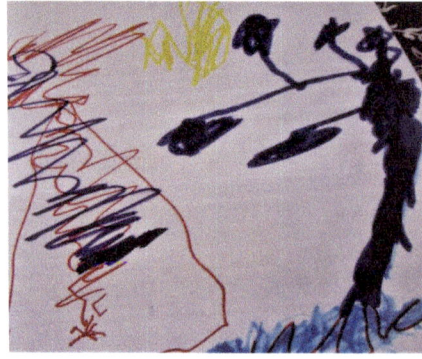
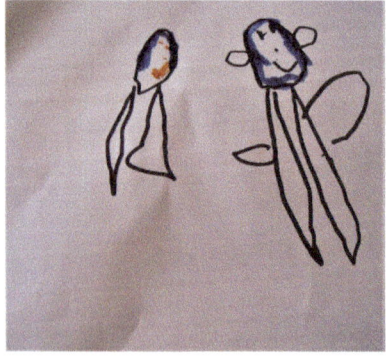

Chart 3.5b Outer genital fighting phase/Stories emerge/Fascination with human figure

loudly that they were just going to have to marry each other. Since that day, I have told my students this story frequently to illustrate four-year-old play and declared that the problem with the world is that girls love boys and boys love trucks!

Outer genital children are incorporating all their previous phases into their sense of self. Children's art represents this as well. Forms begin to have distinct shapes other than circles and are usually meant to represent something, which the child identifies.

With this ability to make recognizable (at least to the child) shapes, making up stories for these graphic images follows their development organically. Usually, during the outer genital phase, a tadpole human figure (DiLeo, 1970, 1973) appears in children's art. A tadpole figure has a circle for a head with facial features. Simple lines come directly out of the circle, two from the side and two from the bottom, representing arms and legs. Often the tadpole figure appears to be floating on the page. Approximately a year after the tadpole figure appears, a torso is added and the human becomes more vertical and grounded on the paper, and other elements start to be added, like the floor, grass or ground, the sky, clouds, the sun, and trees.

Once toddlers have developed through these early stages, they have quite an interesting repertoire of image representations. They freely combine line and form into aesthetically pleasing pieces incorporating shape, color, and placement. I call these *Baby Masterpieces*, and I have nothing else to say about them but that they are a joy to view, so please enjoy.

Dr. Kestenberg's History Books

Part of the KAP is personal books, and I include these here because they involve art, though not necessarily made by a child. A sound intervention employed by Dr. Kestenberg was the use of a personal book made specifically for the child related to an event in their life. For example, if the child requires surgery, or a family member becomes ill or dies, or a parent goes on a business trip and has never been separated from the child, and so on. At CDR, parents who were artists or artistically gifted were drafted to provide the illustrations for Dr. Kestenberg's stories about shared experiences like the arrival of a new baby, weaning, and getting toilet trained, which we would read with the children, especially if someone were going through the experience. If a family expected a new baby imminently, we would read the *New Baby* book with the group and address the about-to-be older-sibling discussing who will be with them when Mommy and Daddy go to the hospital, when they will be able to see the new baby, and where the baby will sleep when brought home. This review helps the child adjust to a big life change by giving them information and group support in a way that is both understandable and digestible.

If a book were made specifically for a child, for example before surgery, Dr. Kestenberg felt it helped the child prepare for the event and support the best possible outcome, and she also explained to the parents that they should

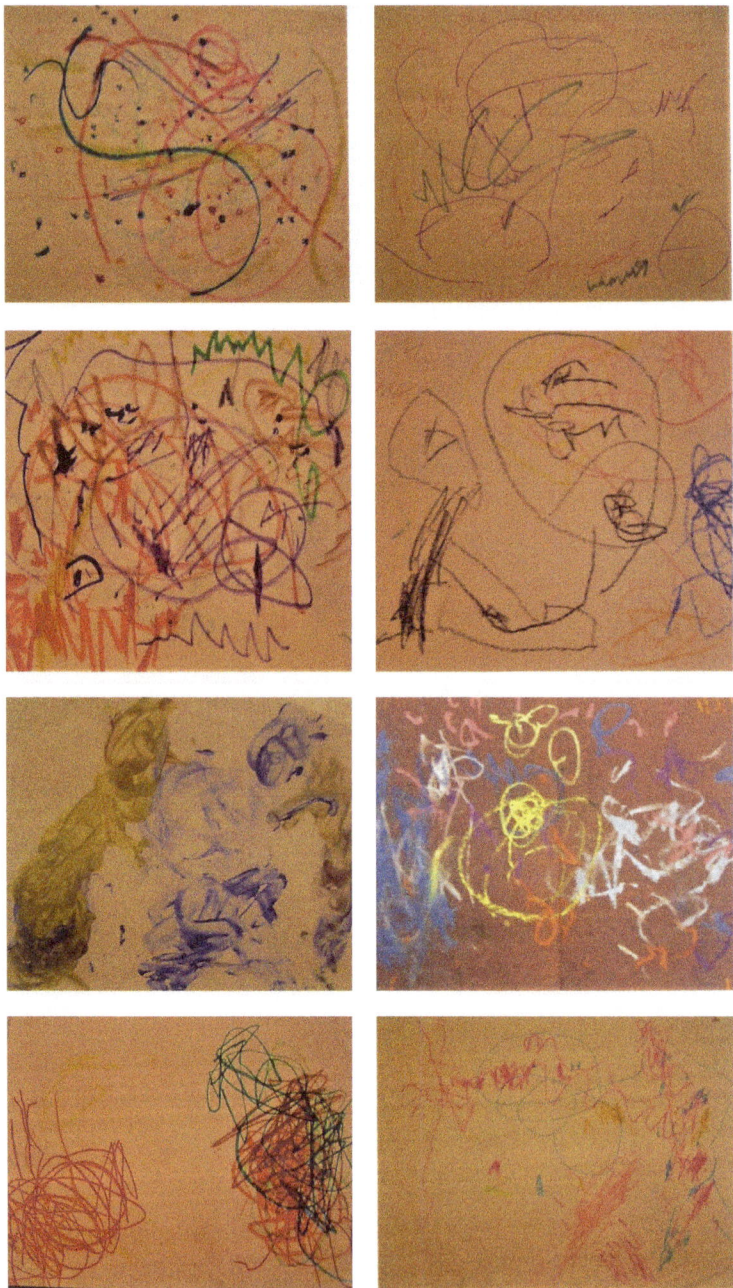

Chart 3.6 Baby masterpieces

keep the book and read it whenever the child requested it. She called it a history book for the child. It told the story of something in the child's history, and by re-reading it, the child can review the event, for better or for worse, and resolve any outstanding questions, concerns, and feelings related to the event.

Sometimes we made books to address behaviors happening at CDR. After Halloween one year, one of the 18-month-old children kept bursting into tears when the older children were playing dress-up. The Mom explained that she had been very scared by people wearing masks when trick-or-treating with her older sibling. So, I made an interactive book where each page had someone wearing a mask, which could be lifted revealing that it was a mommy, daddy, brother, sister, grandparent, or pet. The child stopped crying during dress-up, loved the book, and wanted it to be read often.

Another book was created for the CDR group because one of the older girls was becoming very bossy to the other children, and it was creating problems. As mentioned, the parents stayed with their children at CDR, and stayed till four years old. Dr. Kestenberg felt that children should be with their parents until four and that is when they are ready for school. We talked to the older children about school, telling them that Mommy and Daddy will not be with them and that there are certain expectations in their behavior. We wanted to help this girl stop her bossy behavior by showing her what happens with other children when you are bossy and what happens when you stop being bossy, that is, life gets better. I was often drafted to make these books, but I admit that, as an artist, I am not an illustrator. I relied heavily on magazine and Polaroid® images. Luckily, when it came to making the *bossy* book, one of my interns, Lisa Morrow, volunteered to make the book with simple and whimsical illustrations to which the children could relate. It got the point across.

Linda

Linda was a six-year-old girl with school anxiety. Kindergarten had been only half day, and her neighbor was her teacher and took her to school, so there was not a problem. But first grade became a problem because she was there all day and did not know her teacher since she was a baby. Linda was crying and clinging, would not take the bus, and was having trouble staying in her classroom. She was sad and often burst into tears. Such phobias and anxieties are usually related to unresolved separation issues. Linda's Mom had a chronic medical illness and was hospitalized for large blocks of time when Linda was an infant and toddler. Her Dad was devoted and wonderful, and her grandparents lived nearby and took care of her and her older sister when Mom was in the hospital. But disruption for a child during the early stages of attachment and separation/individuation can be quite traumatic.

At my suggestion, Linda's Mom made a book about her stays in the hospital, with sweet pictures of herself in a hospital gown squatting down to talk to the girls when they visited. We read it together. Linda said to her Mom, "Where's the tree you walked around with?" Her Mom looked at me quizzically, and I explained that I thought

Linda was talking about the IV pole. Her Mom was amazed at Linda's remembering and asking about something from a time when she did not have the language to ask. Her Mom then explained what the "tree" was and about other things that Linda asked about. She also told Linda, very tenderly, that her doctor asked her to not have the girls visit because she became too upset when they left, as did the girls. Her Mom apologized and said she missed them so much but tried her best to get better and get home. They embraced for a long time, and Linda said that she understood. Shortly thereafter, Linda's school phobia faded dramatically, and she was able to take the bus and stay in school for the full day.

Case Study Reflecting Developmental Issues Addressed with the KAP

Victor

Victor was five years old when his mother brought him to me for art therapy. He was a tall boy with thick black hair and striking black eyes, though he did not make eye contact readily. Victor loved art, and the presenting problem, per his mother, was that he was painting only using black, and this concerned her. In the first session, his Mom and younger sister stayed with him, and he did not talk to or look at me. Victor had a beautiful smile with deep dimples but turned away when he smiled. I expressed to his Mom that I did not believe he was seriously depressed and would like to work with him.

The back story is that his parents were Americans living in a socialist country as young adults. They were not successful at conceiving a baby when they decided they wanted to start a family, so decided to adopt. They adopted Victor from an orphanage where he had been placed at birth. He was nine months old and had been swaddled and in a crib for the entire time. When I heard this, I realized that Victor had not progressed through the early movement patterns because of the swaddling. The pediatrician to whom they took Victor after adopting him told them that he was autistic. They did not want to believe this, but I am certain that he must have had infantile depression from lack of contact, holding, and moving. The pediatrician gave them instructions with a strict protocol to follow to make Victor "not autistic." They followed these diligently. Much of it was moving Victor around to help him gain physical mastery of his early movement patterns, which was essential. The other instructions had to do with Victor's eye contact and perceptual field. For example, they held a pencil vertically in front of Victor. After assuring eye contact, they would move the pencil slowly back and forth within an 18-inch range. They would repeat this, and other actions, several times during a session, and then repeat the session every waking hour. I do not know if his parents' great efforts made Victor "not autistic," but they certainly helped him develop movement patterns he missed because of being swaddled, and, importantly, they supported his ability to attach to someone outside of himself, someone who would love and take care of him.

Victor's sister, two years younger, was also adopted while they lived in the socialist nation. However, she was adopted at birth and did not present with the struggles that Victor had. Further, she was stunningly beautiful and had a dazzling personality.

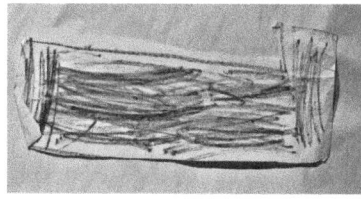
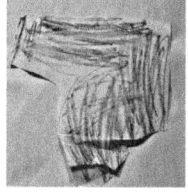
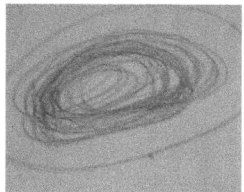

Figures 3.2 Victor's food—French fries, pork chop, spaghetti

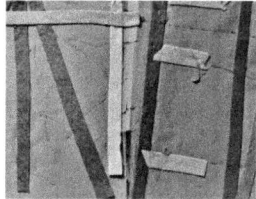
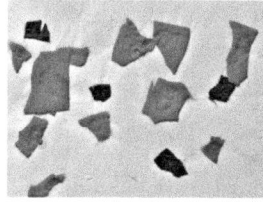
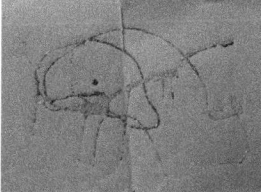

Figures 3.3 Victor's dribbling glue urethral phase

Their Mom and I both realized that she was part of Victor's problem because he would always let her take center stage, so he could fade into the background.

I worked with Victor using a variety of materials and techniques and brought him through the stages of the KAP. We started with drawing. Victor's lines were horizontal and dense and soon became vertical and dense. And the subject matter was always food—French fries, pork chops, spaghetti. I am sure that a baby that was left alone for nine months will always be "hungry" on different levels. His oral and anal art were combined.

Victor's urethral art consisted of his dribbling school glue onto construction paper and then applying pieces of felt or sparkles. The felt was in strips, and so this was like the expanding lines of the urethral phase. He was delighted with this activity, often giggled, and soon Victor's dribbling became more circular, with intention, moving him into the inner genital phase. He began placing smaller pieces of felt onto the paper in a design, which looked like the separate forms that babies draw when forms first appear. And then he used sparkles to outline his circular forms.

Victor's circular forms were soon repeated when he was drawing, but they were not progressing to human form, even though he would often identify them as people. Coincidentally, he was demonstrating dysgraphia at school and was having tremendous difficulty writing numbers and letters. One day, Victor spotted graph paper on my desk that I had been using with an adolescent. He asked if he could use it and proceeded to draw a human form and some numbers with no problem at all. I was astonished. I gave him more graph paper, and human forms appeared again. My thoughts were that the grid pattern helped his brain to organize the space in a way that allowed him to draw at a higher level and write numbers. I suggested to his Mom that she ask his teacher to give him graph paper to write on. With graph paper, Victor was able to write

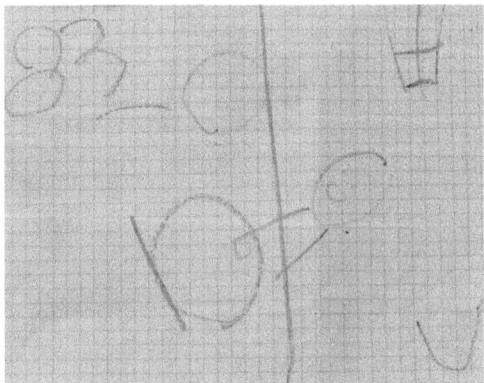

Figure 3.4 Victor drew a person and numbers on graph paper

with no difficulty. I have since shared this with students and professionals so that they could use this with children with dysgraphia. I have since also learned that using a yellow background on a computer screen also supports smoother writing for people with dysgraphia. Another bit of information that I learned along the way and cannot find its source is that when children are ready to read, they start drawing their circles from the top. That was true with Victor, and his Mom thought I was a genius because I told her he was going to start reading soon when he did this.

Victor was soon drawing human forms with all materials and on all paper, moving into the outer genital. They were first tadpoles and then full forms. The arms were always distorted, maybe representing his difficulty with contact. There were many lines drawn on the face, which made it look like he had two sets of eyes or two mouths. Victor told me these were cheeks, and it occurred to me that he was representing dimples, which indicated self-awareness because he had deep dimples. When he iden-tified a figure as himself, there was always a rectangle in the middle of the forehead, which he identified as a bandage. My thoughts were that he felt there was something wrong with him. Victor eventually wanted to cut the figures out, and soon, we made puppets. The bandage appeared on one of the puppet's heads. When asked what the puppet's name was, he said his name was "I don't know." And he named the other puppet with his sister's name. Again, there is a sense of his inadequacies, yet he was developing a stronger sense of self.

One day, Victor asked to paint. I set up an easel and tempera paints for him to use. I enjoyed just watching him paint. He looked like a professional and carefully chose paint and made marks on the page. After doing quite a colorful piece, he put black paint on his brush and covered some of what he had done. Since his presenting problem was that he painted only black paintings, I mentioned this to him. Victor told me very clearly that when he gets to the art station, black might be the only color left. He went on to say that "the black paint is also still thick." When I pushed for an explanation, he expressed that the teachers had added water to other, more popular, colors causing them to be runny, which offended his artist sensibility. Those were not his words but

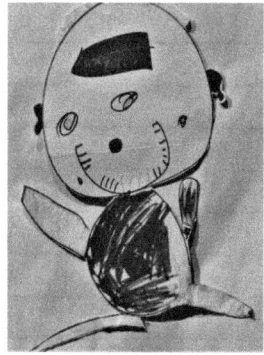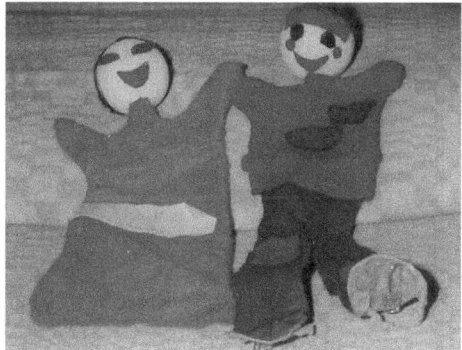

Figures 3.5 Self-representations

his sentiments. I told this to his Mom, who was relieved that he was not depressed. And I have told many parents and students over the years this story to caution against jumping to conclusions. A child may be shy and get to the art station late; a child may enjoy painting and want a pigment that is not watered down; and a child may have some visual problems and enjoy the contrast of black paint on white paper. If a child demonstrated the latter in a session, it would cause me to suggest to parents that they have the child's eyes checked.

*Victor returned to treatment briefly as an adolescent and was attending a special education high school for people with ASD. He was having anxiety and depression, and I assessed him, gave him some relaxation techniques, and we did art. I gave his Mom the name and number of a psychiatrist who was great with teens just because I felt he should be evaluated. I never take adolescent depression lightly. Victor told me that, when he gets overwhelmed or too ADHD, he still sings a few lines from a song to himself that I had taught him to sing when he was a little kid, and that helps him feel better—"*Slow down, you're moving too fast…*"*

Victor's early art in his adolescent treatment was reminiscent of oral and urethral fighting lines. He was experiencing chaotic and intrusive thoughts—he was having trouble with thoughts flowing in and out. I suggested to his Mom that Victor see a cognitive behaviorist who might do biofeedback with him, and a psychiatrist, who might think Victor needs medication, which his parents were, understandably, resistant to. As we progressed in art therapy, his symptoms decreased, and he was more organized. He showed renewed interest in basketball and loved the NY Knicks. He drew pictures of the floor in Madison Square Garden with a grid-like pattern reminiscent of his graph paper drawings. Victor drew a house with a primitive attempt at perspective. However, he explained to me that he often drew a line down the page or across the page to organize the space for himself and remembered that we had used graph paper to do just that. I realized that Victor was able to self-regulate through all the tools he had learned in therapy over the years.

Victor went on to attend a college that had a special program for people with ASD. He joined a support group and demonstrated excellent leadership. In fact, in summers, he worked at a camp for kids with ASD and called me to ask for arts and crafts

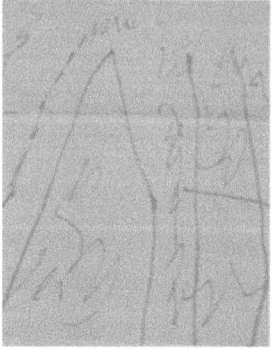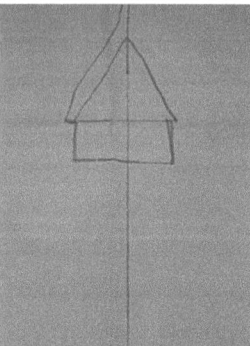

Figures 3.6 Victor's teen art

suggestions with a twist that could help the kids with their emotional issues. "Like you helped me."

Understanding Developmental Interruptions: Application of the KAP to Art of Older Children, Adolescents, and Adults

Just as the KMP can be used as a comprehensive instrument in the context of psychotherapy, teaching, prevention, and intervention, with children as well as adults, so can the KAP. As dance/movement therapists assess movement patterns to support clinical interventions, art therapists can assess art patterns. Both "can provide a tool for enhancing the understanding of the subtle and intricate possibilities for nonverbal relationships" (Loman and Foley, 1996). Both can offer indications of intrapsychic and relational functioning. Both offer practical information about the development of a dynamic formulation as it highlights areas of conflict, pathology, and character expressions as well as areas of harmony and ego strength. Both can be employed to look at relational aspects in the therapeutic context such as bi-directional formation of empathy and attachment, matches and mismatches, and rupture and repair. As the KMP offers a clear and systematic description of an individual's movements, distinguishing between individual preferences and movement in relation to someone else, the KAP offers the same through a review of art. Through this review of patterns in the art, feelings, emotions, and behaviors can be made conscious, described, and eventually experienced differently to affect change. A patient may better understand matches and clashes in relationships, as well as areas of harmony and conflict. The KAP equips the therapist with a tool to better understand developmentally meaningful sequences and themes that appear in the patient's art for the purpose of insight and resolution.

Cases. Mark, Raj, and Kara

Although Mark and Raj are both two years old, and Kara is three, and none are older children, their art illustrates visible disruption as it occurs during a phase.

Mark

Mark's father was morbidly depressed to the point where he took a leave from his job and laid on the couch all day. He was not helping with Mark nor around the house. Consequently, Mark's Mom, who brought him to therapy, was doing the work of both and taking on extra work to pay for daycare because she had no help. I asked Mark to draw Mommy and Daddy. Mark drew Daddy with thick brown anal indulgent lines becoming vertical, anal fighting. He drew Mommy with frantic urethral indulgent rhythms and a great deal of flow, looping back to create primitive form, but he worked over the same area so much that circles eventually appeared—inner genital indulgent. Mommy still reaches out to connect to Daddy, inner genital fighting, offering him support despite all else that she was doing.

To me, this is a perfect representation of this two-year old's world view. Daddy is an unmovable mass, and Mommy is high energy trying to take care of everybody and everything.

Raj

Raj's Dad was arrested for fraud and incarcerated. Raj's Mom had absolutely no idea of what was going on, so when police officers came to the house to arrest him, there was a horrible scene, which Raj witnessed. The next day, Raj drew this image. Urethral indulgent lines flow across the page, and those higher on the page are looping back to create primitive form. In the center of the page, Raj applied heavy lines with an anal

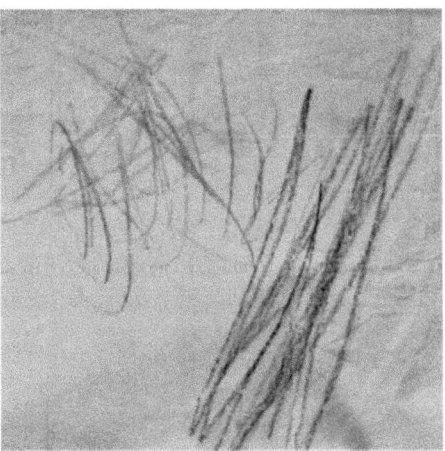

Figure 3.7 Two-year-old Mark's view of his parents

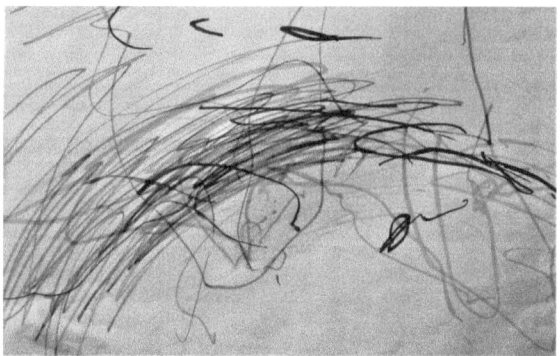

Figure 3.8 Raj's Dad is arrested

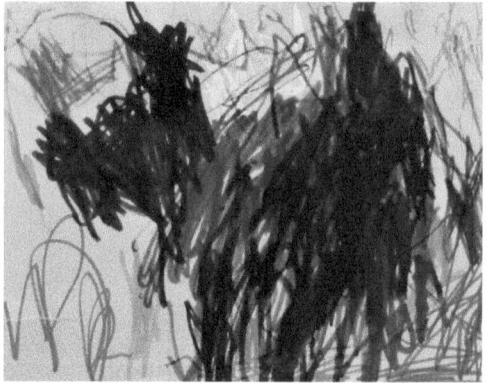

Figure 3.9 Kara's pain

denseness. This whole section arches ominously across the page, anal indulgent, and may represent what Raj was feeling with all these adults yelling and screaming and being upset over him. On the top of the page, there are light oral indulgent lines, perhaps a regression in the moment to try to organize himself and make sense of the scene.

Kara

Kara, at three years old, was manifesting a variety of physical symptoms, including fevers and joint pain. Her art was becoming more and more filled with dense anal lines, and she was covering over and over with color, topped with black. In the bottom left corner of the page, there appears to be a much more delicate cluster of leaf-like forms, urethral indulgent. This form almost looks like it is looking up at the dense mass. Perhaps this represents all the adults examining her, and Kara is the intense mass of pain. Before that time, Kara was drawing lots of forms and circles and demonstrated some talent in art. But this was a regression. Kara was finally diagnosed with lupus.

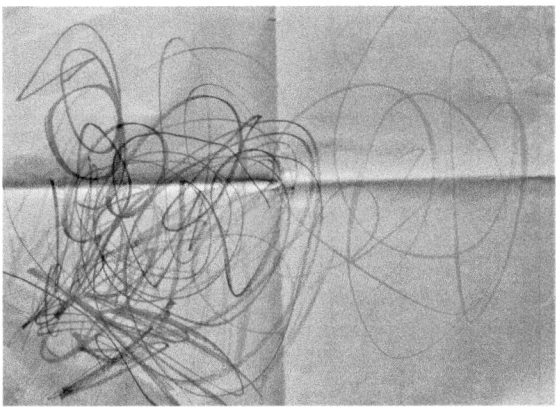

Figure 3.10 Tripp, 6 years old, failure to thrive

Tripp

Tripp was six years old and diagnosed with failure to thrive. Although he was six years old, he was the size of a three-year-old. He was very bright and perceptive with excellent verbal communication skills, belying his small stature. Tripp was also very anxious, as were both his parents. Because he was smart, his parents often discussed matters with him, as if he were an older child or adult. But then, they would apply rules and regulations like parents do with children. This confused Tripp and made him feel out of control. From a young age, Tripp would try to regain control of the world around him by not eating. Tripp would also regress—soiling himself, talking baby talk, and engaging in infantile behavior. Tripp's art is not that of a six-year-old child, but rather of a three-year-old. He clearly had fears of being separated from his Mom, so I feel that part of his regression was so that she would take care of him like a baby. Tripp's drawing has a dense anal base on the right with several circular forms, inner genital indulgent, on top of that. These may be his parents and all the other adults analyzing him and his behavior. My feeling is that the circular form on the right is Tripp. This form is separated and individuated from the rest, yet there is a connector line, inner genital fighting, going in and out of the mass, possibly representing Tripp with both his fears of separation and his manipulating them all.

Jenna

Jenna was a nine-year-old girl with severe asthma, who was in the hospital often. The hospital staff were beginning to suspect abuse but had no hard evidence to call child protective services. Jenna's drawing looks distressed. There are thick anal lines coming from the chimney, which can indicate stress in the home. There are clothes on the line. Maybe this was Jenna's way of hanging out the family's dirty laundry for the hospital staff to see. But the repetitive dotting of the raindrops, oral fighting, often indicate fear of separation. Even though children may be abused in their homes, they still fear separation from their parents, who may be the abusers. Children may be frightened because

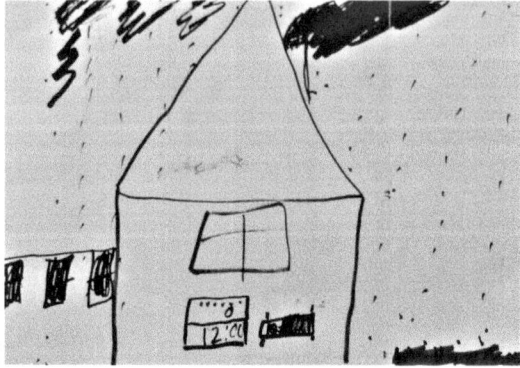

Figure 3.11 Jenna, nine years old, with chronic asthma

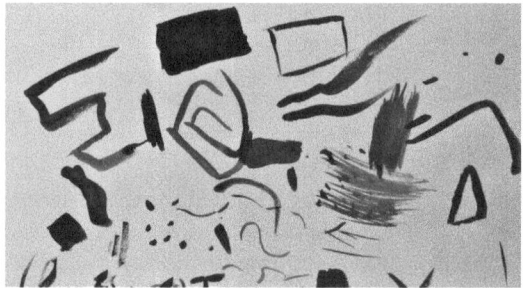

Figure 3.12 11-year old Brian's language that girls cannot understand.

they are threatened by their parents—"if you tell anyone, they will take you away and put me in jail"—or they may simply be frightened that what is out there may be worse than their current situation.

Brian

Brian was 11 years old when his Mom brought him for art therapy. He was diagnosed with ADHD, and was becoming increasingly defiant. Brian was in a gifted class, which was all boys, and he and his friends were becoming increasingly hostile towards women and girls. My sense is that they were in the throes of puberty and could not make sense of their feelings. Brian's art was typical of his age with lots of cartoon-like images and humorous, though dark, stories to accompany them. After a defiant incident with me, his teacher, and an older girl who babysat him, I was pushing Brian to talk about what he might think is going on with him and "girls." After ignoring me for several minutes, Brian took paper and drew this image that includes oral fighting dotting, anal indulgent denseness, urethral fighting zigzags, and some non-circular forms, outer genital indulgent. When I inquired what it was, Brian told me that it was a language

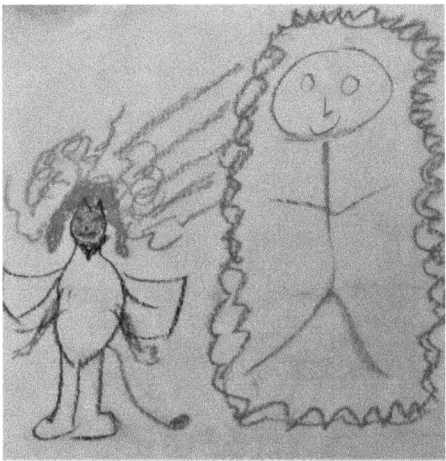

Figure 3.13 Kenny's rapprochement dance with his Mom

that I could not understand because I am a girl. My sense was that his regressed art was pointing to a time that he did not feel understood. It also happened to be a time when his Mom returned to work full-time.

Kenny

Kenny was 16 years old and considered himself Goth. He and his friends were into on-line role playing, and their story lines were dark. This is perfectly typical for adolescents to explore and indentify with beliefs and philosophies that are different from their parents. His Mom was a single Mom, and Kenny was an only child. They were almost too close. His Mom was tolerant of his behavior, except when it was inter-fering with his grades. In this drawing, Kenny shows his Mom after a poor report card. His Mom looks blankly from inside the circular form, inner genital. The border of the circle is made with urethral fighting lines. Toddlers often identify this as their signed name—putting their stamp on the art. My feeling is that this circle is Kenny defining his mother's identity—this stick figure with a static smile and blank eyes. Yet, he feels like she is staring at him with anger about his poor report card and sees him as a devil. Kenny looks more like a cat than a devil with dense anal lines around his head and inner genital circles floating above. This looks like a dance between the anal stage of control and the inner genital stage of containment, and this is the dance that Kenny and his Mom do. There are also many connector lines, inner genital fighting, going back and forth between them.

Todd

Todd was 22 years old, and gay. He was not open about it and was in a committed relationship, so he wanted to tell his parents. He asked me for help, and I had him

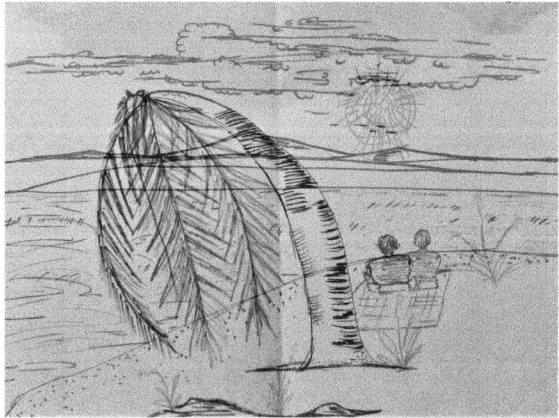

Figure 3.14 Todd anticipating telling his parents that he is gay

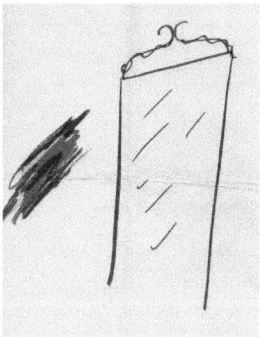

Figure 3.15 Ronit gets no reflection from her mother

draw his relationship with his boyfriend. The sun is often understood as a symbol of paternal authority. The seagulls around the sun look like urethral fighting signature lines. Todd may be representing his explaining his identity to his Dad. The tree looks like a weeping tree. Perhaps this is how Todd expects his Mom to react. The tree is surrounded by oral indulgent little short strokes, attaching to mother, and oral fighting dotting, separating from mother both on land and sea.

Ronit and Susan

Ronit and Susan both had narcissistic mothers. Much of the work of their therapy was to stop trying to please their mothers and embracing their separate identity to have better adult relationships.

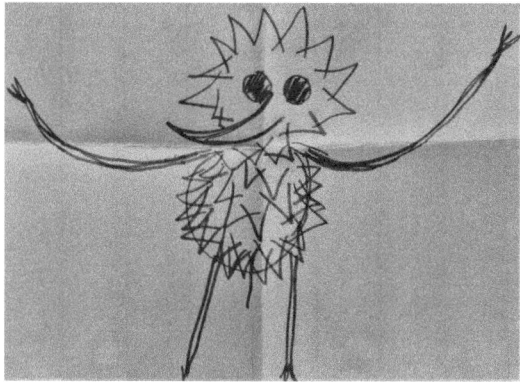

Figure 3.16 Susan's mother

Ronit

Ronit, 32, was a struggling artist. She had four older brothers, all of whom were accomplished professionals in their fields. Apparently, they satisfied her mother's narcissistic needs, and her mother reminded Ronit of that regularly. Ronit drew this image of herself looking into a mirror. She is a dense anal indulgent blob, but she is becoming vertical, anal fighting, and leaning towards the mirror, but there is no reflection. Ronit quickly identified the mirror as her mother, who never reflects back to her.

Susan

Susan, 28, was finishing up graduate school and working hard on her relationship with her boyfriend. Susan's mother was narcissistic and diagnosed with schizoaffective disorder. When Susan was two years old, her sister was born. Immediately after the birth, her mother was unstable and was psychiatrically hospitalized for six months. Susan's father was inadequate and disengaged from both girls. Susan and I both agreed that she was as mentally healthy as she was because she was raised by her loving aunt and uncle who lived in the same building. But much of her time was spent trying to analyze issues with her mother. During one session, Susan said she felt anxious and wanted something to hold. I gave her some modeling clay, which is an anal material, to work with her hands while she lay on the couch. At the end of the session, we processed it. It looked like a blue hourglass. Susan looked at it and said, "Look at this. This is my cold blue mother with no arms to hold me and no legs to take me anywhere with her." She was sad and put the piece down. When she looked at her hands, they were blue stains from the clay. Susan laughed and said, "Look at this! I can't get rid of her. She's under my skin!"

That piece of art helped Susan move away from that two-year-old child, who was abandoned in the anal stage to a stage where she felt more separate from her mother and her mother's mental illness. This rendering of her mother dominates with urethral fighting lines, perhaps identifying her mother, but their sharpness keeps her mother protected from everyone else's identity and protects her narcissism. The eyes look sad, and Susan was trying to be more accepting of her mother's illness. But the long-pointed nose indicated her mother's intrusiveness and tendency to hurt them with words and actions if they failed to meet her narcissistic needs. The arms are open for an embrace but look limp, and that nose might discourage coming closer, and the legs are weak looking—not much better than the clay hourglass with no legs to take her anywhere.

Cass

Cass, 33, was a working artist. Her husband was dying, and she used her art to process something that was very hard for her to talk about. Cass's urethral indulgent lines flow across the page, running, running. Time was running out. There are little pockets, inner genital indulgent, with repetitive designs, which I felt Cass made to try to contain and organize the process of dealing with her husband's death. In the upper left-hand corner, there is an eye because Cass was trying to watch this journey and

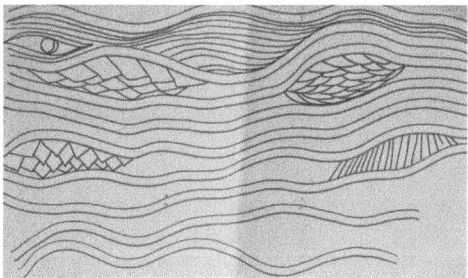

Figure 3.17 Time flowing away

decide what she wanted to do. Eventually, Cass left her full-time job and did contract work to be more available to her husband during his treatments. And finally, she took leave from her job, and they traveled around the country together enjoying their last few months together.

Carlos

Carlos, 46, was a recovering addict and was HIV+. He attended Narcotics Anonymous (NA) meetings faithfully. But he had unprotected sex with women he met there stating that if you have unprotected sex with someone you meet at NA, then you are probably HIV+. I tried to convince him of the flaws in this thought process, but Carlos was unmoved. Carlos had trafficked drugs for many years of his adult life and used IV drugs since he was a young adolescent. He reported stories of wanting to shoot himself or jump out of the window of the hotel where he was waiting for drug dealers to buy his stuff, which was one of the reasons he stopped using. Carlos had a congenital disorder in his bones that caused him tremendous pain and may have been one of the reasons he started using drugs. While Carlos had a daily routine that was calm, his art indicates chaotic and disorganized thinking. He always drew quickly with a variety of lines and forms, anal, urethral, inner genital, and pointed things out like a story, outer genital fighting. But there was never a sense of cohesion that one might get from a four year old telling a story about their art. Carlos took his methadone and HIV medicine but did not otherwise take good care of his health, eating poorly, not exercising, and only sleeping a few hours a night. Perhaps his images reflect his deteriorating physical and mental condition.

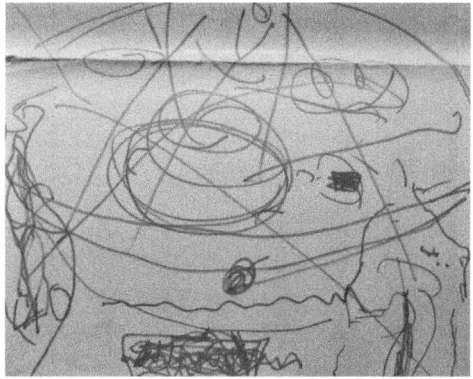

Figure 3.18 Carlos story of drug use

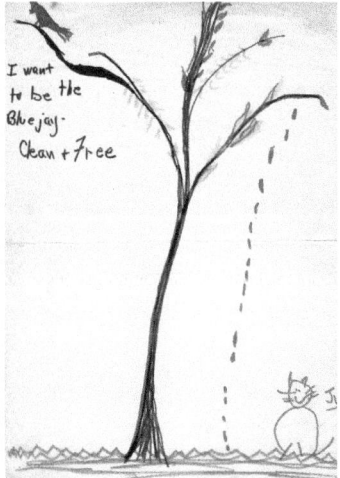

Figure 3.19 I want to be free as the blue jay

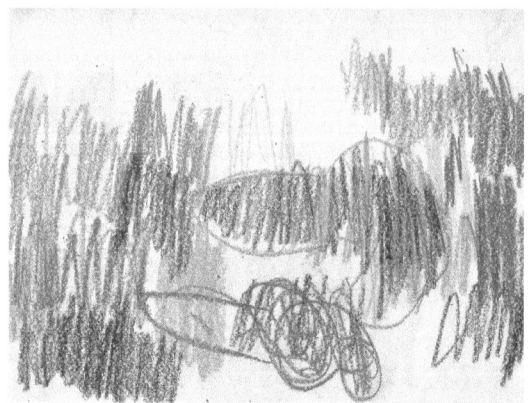

Figure 3.20 Earnie, 68, lived in an institution since birth

Evelyn

Evelyn was 50 and a professional musician, as was her husband, Sid. When they came to me as a couple, Sid said he wanted to work on their relationship, and Evelyn said she wanted me to make Sid stop smoking pot. They had a very symbiotic relationship, and Sid was fine with that. But Evelyn felt smothered and wanted some emotional separation. She drew herself inside three boxes with the words "I can't breathe" written on the outside. After a while, she drew this image. It is a bit ironic that she stated that she wants to be free as a bird, yet has her cat, Jim, who goes after birds, waiting at the bottom of the tree. However, her raindrops, oral fighting dotting, drip down into urethral fighting lines representing the grass. Evelyn wants the separation and to proclaim her separate identity.

Earnie

Earnie, 68, lived in a large state institution for people with developmental disabilities since birth. He had significant cognitive deficits, poor vision, and no language. Earnie was not usually interested in communicating unless he wanted to make his basic needs known. His art resembles that of a three-year-old, including lines and form. It is likely that Earnie's level of cognition was that of a toddler.

4 Theories of Human Development and Developmental Art Theories

How does understanding art developmentally help us when we look at patient artwork?

Knowledge of children who are typically developing and their developmental art helps us better understand what is going on when observing a typical behavior or when seeing indicators of pathology, trauma, or organicity, for example, in children's art. When using a developmental framework in treatment, the therapist takes the patient's personal developmental history into consideration. This model supports the therapist's insight and understanding of: how and why presenting problems came about; what the diagnostic indicators are; how treatment should proceed; and what materials would optimally be used to support goals and good treatment outcomes.

Mahler's (1968) discussion of separation/individuation and rapprochement describes how significant this time of life is for healthy ego development and offers valuable information into the person's attachment and separation issues. My experience has been that this transition from attachment to separation, and the accompanying rapprochement dance, plays out as one transitions from one stage to the next throughout life and will always replay during those transitional times. For example, when a child enters kindergarten or when a latency-aged child goes through puberty and becomes an adolescent, they may have tantrums because the world feels out of control just as it did when they were three years old. When leaving college and entering the job force, when getting married, when starting a family, or when on the verge of retirement, the ever-developing human may demonstrate emotional lability because the world that has been in their control for so long is about to be out of their control, just as it was when they were three. Understanding how a patient went through the first attachment and separation can shed light on their ego strengths, as well as their relationship with their mother—all useful information in treatment. And being sensitive to this tendency to repeat rapprochement during transitions in a patient's life offers therapists a valuable tool in seeing the whole picture of the patient before them. In fact, Mahler's (1968) discussion of separation/individuation and rapprochement has been applied to the understanding of Borderline Personality Disorder (Horner, 1979).

The theories of human development that offer a rounded perspective are Freud's (1905) psychosexual and drive theory, Piaget's (1936) theory of cognition, and Erikson's (1950) psychosocial theory. It is reasonable to consider all these aspects of development to get a full picture. We grow and develop through drives; we experiment and learn through our cognition; we are social beings starting from family throughout life. Erikson was among the first theorists to outline stages of life beyond adolescence into adulthood.

Many of the pioneers of art therapy, and other childhood specialists, offer frameworks concerning the development of children's art. These developmental art theories from the following authors' classic texts are reviewed and synthesized in this chapter (appear here in alphabetical order):

Joseph H. DiLeo's (1970) *Young Children and their Drawings*
    (1973) *Children's Drawings as Diagnostic Aids*
    (1977) *Child Development: Analysis and Synthesis*
    (1983) *Interpreting Children's Drawings*
Howard Gardner's (1980) *Artful Scribbles: The Significance of Children's Drawings*
Rhoda Kellogg's (1967) *Analyzing Children's Art*
Myra Levick's (1998) *See What I'm Saying: What Children Tell Us Through their Art*
Viktor Lowenfeld's and W.L. Brittain's (1957) *Creative and Mental Growth*
Judith Rubin's (1984) *Child Art Therapy*

At the end of this chapter, there is a chart representing these authors, and it includes Judith Kestenberg, to offer a comparison and better understanding of the different stages they define across the developmental continuum.

I want to acknowledge the contributions to developmental art theory by Viktor Lowenfeld. Although his work was based on his experience as an art teacher, not an art therapist, his philosophy was therapeutic in nature. He observed thousands of typically and atypically developing children creating thousands of pieces of artwork. His intrinsic understanding of unfolding human development is keen. These observations led to his developmental descriptors, which are valid and solid in their representation of age groups to this day. Lowenfeld understood how important making art was to developing children and observed deviations from what was typical in the art. And he wrote it all down, with wisdom, for future generation to learn from. The reaches of Lowenfeld's (1987) therapeutic insight may be seen in his work *Therapeutic Aspects of Art Education*, which was a model for how art education can move into the realm of therapy with sensitivity and careful guidance. This was a chapter in the third edition of *Creative and Mental Growth* (1975), which was removed by Brittain after Lowenfeld's death and before the fourth edition. But Elinor Ulman, a pioneer of art therapy and an editor of the *American Journal of Art Therapy*, rescued it from the editor's floor and gave art therapists the gift of reprinting it, with permission, in the journal. In her introduction to the reprint of the chapter, Ulman tells Lowenfeld's story and this history of the chapter. Regarding his analysis of the usual evolution of a series of developmental stages of children's art, she states, "…his terminology and his ideas about the psychological implications of the various stages gained widespread credence" (p. 112).

Understanding the Art Through a Developmental Lens

Early Childhood

Freud (1905) describes the *oral*, *anal*, and *phallic* as the stages of early childhood development. These define the areas of libidinal cathexis in the infant and young child. The work of the oral stage is taking in through the mouth—eating and tasting the world. The work of the anal stage is elimination. This obviously refers to defecating, but the toddler in the anal stage also "eliminates" by spitting out, throwing, or pushing away things in their environment. And the area of cathexis for the phallic stage is the genital region. Children are aware of sensations and curious about where babies come from. Some young children engage in masturbatory activity, such as rocking themselves on top of a toy or stuffed animal.

Piaget (1936) describes typical cognitive growth and development. The earliest phase of cognition is the *Sensorimotor Stage*. During this time, the infant learns through their body experiences by moving and through senses. The baby does not yet internally represent events or think conceptually, yet schemata are being constructed. The toddler is in the stage called *Preoperational*. This stage is characterized by language development and other forms of representation. This is a time of rapid conceptual development, and reasoning is prelogical. The child's thinking is dominated by egocentrism, and in this stage, the child is both individuating and learning through manipulating and interacting with the environment.

Erikson's (1950) early stages of psychosocial theory are *Trust vs. Mistrust*, *Autonomy vs. Doubt/Shame*, and *Initiative vs. Guilt*. Erikson's model reflects a continuum from positive to negative for each stage to describe social and emotional growth for the child. As the child interacts with the world, their experiences will mold who they become. Erikson's model is like building blocks in that each stage provides a basis for the subsequent, and so on. If a baby is loved and cared for, trust will develop, allowing an optimum path towards autonomy as separation and individuation occur, and the child develops a strong sense of self. If this unfolds within good parameters, then the child will be able to take initiative when making choices and interacting with the environment. In the stage of *Trust vs. Mistrust*, a rudimentary sense of trust establishes the groundwork for mutuality and the capacity for giving to others. Mistrust will emerge when the infant develops a profound sense of discomfort and danger. In the stage of *Autonomy vs. Doubt/Shame*, the child must risk breaching the trustful relationship with the mother to progress and attain autonomy. This supports healthy ego development and determines free choice and self-restraint. A prominence of *Initiative* over *Guilt* results in adaptive ego quality of purpose, or courage to pursue valued goals uninhibited by fear of punishment.

Since the previous chapter thoroughly explores the significance of early childhood art per the KAP, that theory will not be addressed here. When reviewing developmental art theory most of the theorists stress the importance of scribbling in art development. While they do not all assign particular significance to the subtle differences within the scribbles, each defines the stage as a clear and necessary stage.

Kellogg (1967), a preschool teacher, feels all the stages of art development are universal and sequential. All children draw circles, which she identifies as suns and mandalas. Kellogg calls the earliest phase the *Scribbling Stage* (ages two to three) and presents hundreds of examples of art created during this stage from children of various cultural and ethnic backgrounds. She feels there is a strong visual component to the development of scribbles. Although she delineates 20 *Basic Scribbles* that appear by the age of two, she does not necessarily assign these specifically to behaviors or months of life. Kellogg relates *Placement Patterns*, her next stage, to the development of the art for children from two to four years of age. Children of this age do not have the eye-hand coordination to accurately represent what they are trying to, so Kellogg feels that they use placement on the page to express the idea. These *Placement Patterns* eventually lead to the early representation of more than one form evolving into the *Two Shape Stage* (three to four years). Kellogg identifies these shapes as either *Outline* or *Implied*. The *Outline* shape is as it sounds—the form is drawn and is an outline, usually a circle, oblong, or irregular rectangle and often with an "X" shape included. The *Implied* shape, or *Emergent Diagram*, is usually a collection of shapes near each other on the page around which one might draw a line to create a shape of a circle, square, or triangle.

Lowenfeld and Brittain(1957) also calls this the *Scribbling Stage*. An art educator, Lowenfeld defines three levels of this in a developmental continuum—*Disordered* to *Controlled* to *Named*. While he acknowledges the importance of scribbling in development, he places the age parameters for this stage as from 18 months to four years of ages, which implies anything before this time has little significance. *Disordered* scribbles (18 months) are random in placement and direction, and Lowenfeld feels they are more of a kinesthetic experience than an art experience because there is little visual or fine motor control. While *Controlled* scribbles (two years) look like disordered ones, the child has more visual control and the ability to keep the drawing implement on the paper. Longitudinal and circular marks are created by repeated motions. *Named* scribbles (three-and-one-half to four years) demonstrate an approach to the drawing task that reflects the child's personality, that is with intention and boldly or timidly presenting repetitive stereotypes. Children of this age place their scribbles purposely. At this point, the artmaking has transformed from kinesthetic to imaginative thinking. They relate the marks they make to things that are known to them. Color is insignificant. In fact, black on white or white on black may be preferential because of the contrast it offers to developing visual coordination.

Rubin (1984), an art therapist, gives the early part of this stage the title of *Manipulating*. While scribbling is essential during this phase, she describes that manipulating and experimenting with materials for a sensory experience is the primary work of this stage. Rubin's next stage is *Forming*. The young child matures into this stage with more cognition and eye-hand coordination and intentionally creates forms. This leads naturally into Rubin's *Naming* stage. She ponders whether this stage is a result of adults asking what the child has made or simply that the child has more control and ownership and so names the forms.

Gardner (1980), a child psychologist, and Levick (1998), an art therapist, give us models which relate the development of scribbles and graphic images to burgeoning cognition. Gardner equates scribbling to babbling suggesting that without babbling, we do not develop speech patterns and without scribbling, we do not develop patterns for graphic representation. Levick echoes this and offers 18 months to two-and-a-half years as the age for this phase. She calls this the *Babble-Scribble Stage Sequence.* Similarly, as Gardner declares that the toddler develops a *Romance with Forms* in art when labeling and classifying in language development, Levick describes this language/art relationship in her *Word-Shape Stage Sequence* from two-and-a-half to four years of age. Gardner expands on the *Romance with Forms* by classifying two groups of young artists as *Patterners* and *Dramatists*. Both groups are delighted with the creation of form on paper and satisfied with their results but have different motivation. *Patterners* approach drawing with the intention of creating a named subject. Sometimes, they even name it after the fact because it looks like something when they are done. *Dramatists* set out to tell a story with their art.

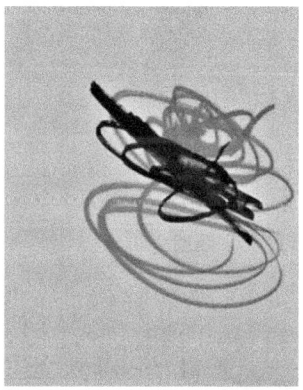 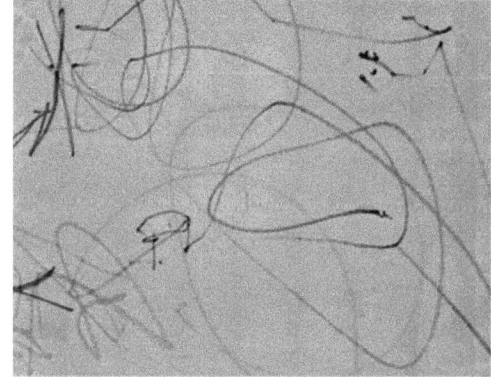

Figure 4.1a Patterner's butterfly   *Figure 4.1b Dramatist's* going to the beach

My observations of two- and three-year old children is that there is a true romance with forms. Their own imagery goes back and forth from art representation to verbal expression as their ability to charmingly represent form in art and describe the world around them grows. At this age, my youngest son called penguins "snowman ducks" and waving flags "uppa yeah yeahs." My three-year-old grandson calls toy trucks that have no batteries "statue trucks" or "hand push" because they stand still and do not move on their own. Children at this age are starting to better understand what is going on both within and outside of themselves and are creating relevant imagery and integrating it cognitively and for problem solving. When watching a documentary on wildfires with my nephew when he was three, he remarked that they should cut the trees down around the fire so it cannot spread to those trees, therefore, slowing the fire's spread. That is exactly where they start, but at this age, he had the ability to have the image of the trees and the fire so clearly that he could offer a solution to a problem.

DiLeo (1970, 1973, 1977, 1983) is a physician and observes development from a medical perspective. He wrote about the child's behavior and intellectual development as it relates to artmaking. He observed that children draw what is important to them—people, animals, houses, trees. Children draw some of what is known about the object because they draw an inner, not an optical, reality. They draw what they remember of their perceptions at the time that they are drawing.

While DiLeo's contributions are valuable, once again, there is a recognition that early scribbling is essential but not significant as can be seen in his title for this phase—*Unrecognizable Representations.* He does believe that scribbling in visual representations is akin to babbling in speech. I agree with him and have found that children will go through the developmental stages regardless of their age when they first draw. For example, a child who has not been exposed to art materials until the age of five will first scribble and then quickly progress to line and form but will progress through identified stages. Similarly, when young children are sitting and drawing a series of pieces, I have seen progress through the stages unfold through the series.

DiLeo offers a model that outlines the development of the human figure in art. He assigned the term *Tadpole*, sometimes called the cephalopod, to describe the earliest human representations, which are circles with the arms and legs coming out from the circle, often drawn on an angle and with a rudimentary face. The *Tadpole* is a giant leap forward for the child artist. DiLeo states that the child has drawn an adult, not a child. He further states that children usually draw people other than themselves, and this indicates a strong ego. DiLeo discusses the young child's fascination with the belly button, fantasizing that perhaps this is where babies come out, and belly buttons are often featured on people drawn by young children. He does not offer strict age parameters for his stages, but rather sees these stages following each other in a sequence. His next step in this sequence is the *Transitional Stage* during which the trunk appears, followed by *Full Face with Progressive Addition of Body Parts.*

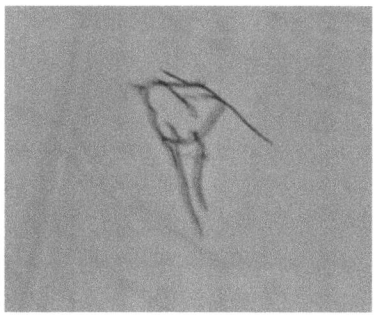

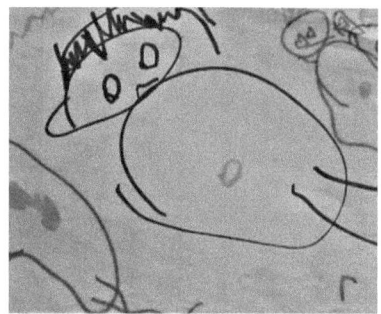

Figure 4.2a A very early tadpole

Figure 4.2b Fascination with belly buttons

Lowenfeld identifies the human form as appearing during the *Named Scribble Stage*; Rubin states that human forms emerge during the *Representing* stage; Gardner discusses *Tadpoles as Things* and relates it to the child's awareness of the importance of humans in their life and an increase in the child's sense of self; and Kellogg states that the human form appears as an *Implied Diagram* and as a *Placement Pattern*.

The previous chapter was devoted to the early art, mostly called scribbles across the board, as classified through the KAP. Therefore, a variety of tadpoles are presented here for a delightful viewing experience.

Childhood: Preschool and School Years

Freud defines this phase of development as the *Latency Period* (age five to the onset of puberty). This refers to a latency in sexual drive. If a child between five years of age and the onset of puberty is overly interested in or preoccupied with sexuality, this is a red flag. However, this is not a latency stage for learning and social/emotional growth. In fact, it is a rich and active time in these areas. Sexuality yields to a safer form of expression, and personality is firmly established during this time.

Piaget describes this stage as *Concrete Operational* when a child's cognitive growth is extraordinary. It is a time when a child learns to read, write, and understand basic mathematics. Children's brains are like sponges, and they absorb so much of what is going on around them. They are curious and energetic. Children develop the ability to apply logical thought to concrete problems. They make judgment based on reasoning. There is a liberation from egocentrism, which comes primarily from social interaction with other children.

Erikson defines this stage as *Industry vs. Inferiority*. It is a time of great industry on the child's part. The child's successes contribute to a positive sense of industry, while failures result in feelings of inadequacy and inferiority. It is also the time when the child enters the world outside of family,

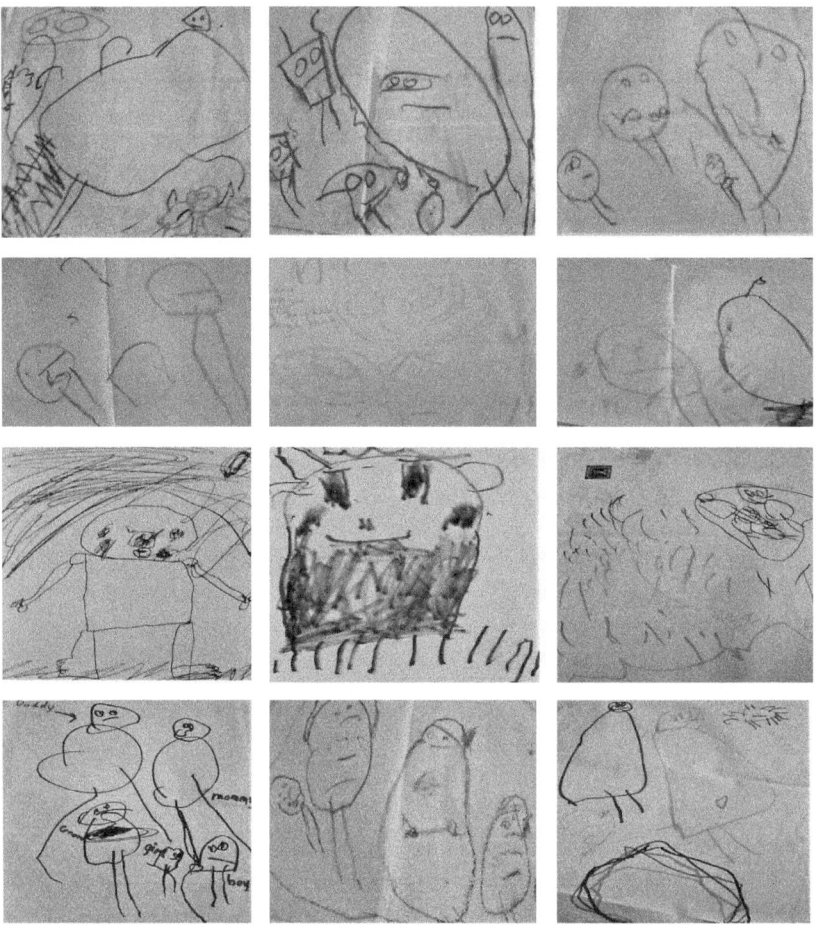

Chart 4.1 Tadpoles and assorted early humans

as they enter school. And their natural interest in everything is enhanced by their interactions with peers and kind, caring adults. During this phase, the child tends to sublimate sexual intrusiveness and re-route social initiative into a skillful activity.

The art of preschool and school-aged children is natural and joyful. Their use of color and form is uninhibited and expressive. They are unafraid of experimenting with art materials, techniques, and supplies, and if they are, an art therapist might suspect the child has issues. And by understanding what appears typically in children's art, an art therapist can identify if children have issues from indicators in the art that are not typical.

Kellogg identifies the *Design Stage* as occurring from three to five years of age. As children mature during these years, Kellogg's basic scribbles, placement patterns, shapes, suns, and circles begin to come together aesthetically into what she identifies as *Combines* and *Aggregates*. Kellogg places five-year-old children in the stage of *Early Pictorialism*. Once human form has appeared in children's art, Kellogg states that the next pictures to emerge are animals, buildings, vegetation, and transportation. These follow her patterns of emerging diagrams, and she feels they are works of art. During the *Later Pictorial Stage*, from five to seven years of age, children are learning many new symbol systems in school, learning to read, write, and do arithmetic and are very much influenced by adults. Consequently, the cognitive development of this stage results in more organization and additions in the art. The adult influence and social/emotional development of this stage result in art that may not be naturally organic for the child and may reflect this influence. Kellogg is opposed to adult influence and rails against formal art education because they both squash this organic art development. She cites stick figures, smiley faces, full lips, and hearts as something an adult might impose onto children's ideas of what should be in their art. She even includes *Houses that most teachers would like* (Kellogg, 1967, p. 156) to emphasize her point that children's beautiful natural art is compromised by their desire to satisfy adults. Not surprisingly, Kellogg's *Final Stage* of art development is self-taught art from seven years of age on. She regrets that children identified as gifted artists at a young age often lose that natural talent when exposed to formal art education.

Lowenfeld believed evidence of aesthetic, social, physical, intellectual, and emotional growth is reflected in the art of children. He breaks the preschool through school-aged years into three categories. Children from four to seven years of age are in the *Pre-schematic Stage*, from seven to nine years of age are in the *Schematic Stage*, and from nine to 11 years of age are in the stage of *Dawning Realism*.

During the *Pre-schematic Stage*, forms are solidly part of children's drawings and start to make more sense to adult judgment. Rudimentary symbols are solid in the child's repertoire, and it is during this stage that the human form appears. Lowenfeld feels that children draw human forms first because they have a relationship with what they intend to represent. Representational symbols change constantly. What children draw is their perception, not from visual stimuli nor mental conception. Art becomes a communication

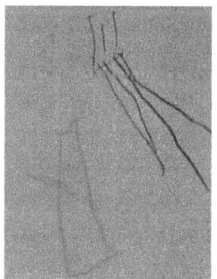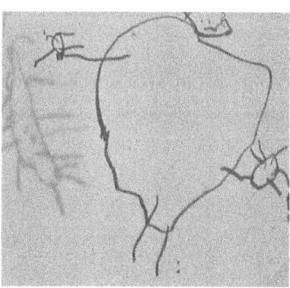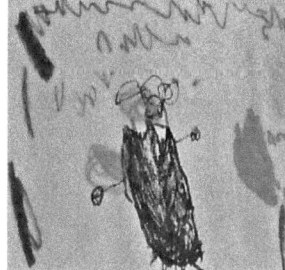

Figures 4.3 Emerging schemas

with the self. The child is engaged in exploration. Spatial relationships are according to emotional significance. Color is insignificant next to form.

The *Schematic Stage* continues with recognizable representation of symbols. As Lowenfeld calls them, *Schema* are represented. A *Schema* is a form that is continuously repeated until a collective expression emerges. The *Schema* is altered when special meaning is conveyed. Pictures may contain people, houses, trees, or objects in a story. A baseline appears, and composition and color become more important to the child. However, all the players and objects may be placed straight across that line because a child of this age does not yet have a sense of perspective and proportion. There is a gap between sky and ground, which is typical.

A Mom brought her seven-year-old daughter, Hazel, to me for art therapy because she was concerned something was happening on the bus to upset her because every time the little girl drew a school bus, she covered it over. Hazel was not otherwise exhibiting any symptoms of anxiety or depression. When she entered my art room, I asked Hazel to draw a school bus for me. Hazel drew a perfectly typical drawing for her age. She drew the groundline in black for a road and the skyline in blue. Hazel drew a delightful looking school bus in yellow and put children's faces in the window, and a driver in the front. She looked at her drawing for a moment and then took a blue crayon and started to cover it over. I asked her to stop and explain to me what she was doing. Hazel's Mom was an artist and had directed Hazel to make the sky meet the ground. However, because of her perception at her level of cognition, Hazel could not successfully make the sky meet the ground without covering over the school bus. She did not yet have the cognitive ability to color around the bus as an older child could do. I suggested to Hazel that she just keep on making art the way she knows how, and I suggested, with good humor, to Hazel's relieved Mom that she not interfere with her daughter's artmaking.

Lowenfeld's last stage for children this age is *Dawning Realism*. Lowenfeld also calls this the *Gang Age* because it is a time of great social interaction with interactions represented in the art, and children's artmaking is influenced by their peers. Sexual distinctions emerge in the art. Girls tend to add animals to their repertoire and enhancements, like hearts and flowers. Boys tend to draw vehicles—cars, trucks, planes, tanks, ships. During this time, children's art skills grow, especially as they move towards the end of this stage when their cognition is developing a sense of spatial depth, perspective, and proportion. However, sometimes art in this stage is somewhat rigid because the child is still in the stage of concrete operations. Color becomes important. Lowenfeld identifies a phenomenon during this stage called *Folding Out*. Children in this stage still very much think of themselves as the center of the world, so they will represent the *Schema* from their point of view. *Xray* drawings are typical at this age, that is, the child represents inside and outside at once, so the viewer can see the outside of a house, as well as all the people and activities going on inside the house. However, *Xray* drawings done by an older child or adult may indicate psychosis.

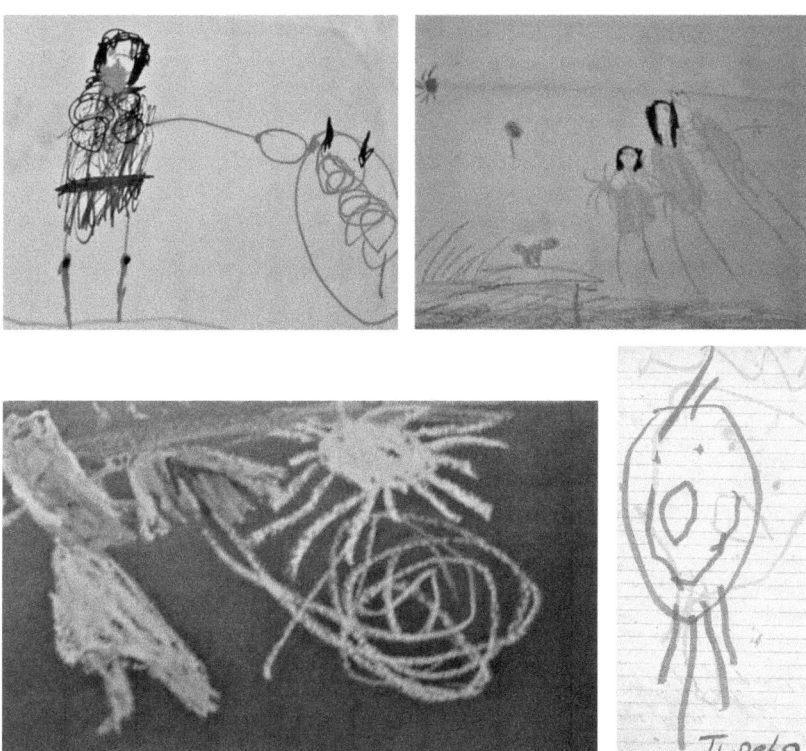

Figure 4.4 Schematic art: (Clockwise) Dorothy and Toto, friends playing, a dog, girl
dancing

Rubin describes the next four stages in her sequence: *Representing,
Containing, Experimenting,* and *Consolidating.* These stages include preschool
and school-aged children. When in the *Representing* stage, the child begins
to bring together the forms that incubated in the three previous stages of
Manipulating, Forming, and *Naming.* These forms are recognizable to them but
may not be to adults. Early human figures appear in this stage, and Rubin
identifies them as *cephalopods,* another term commonly used to identify
early human forms, and as the child goes through this stage, additional facial
features appear.

Rubin's next stage is *Containing.* The child has more self-awareness in this
stage and is more confident in their art. They begin to include more lines,
forms, and details in their composition and fill in space and color. Children
of this age take pride staying in the lines because that is like the way that they
are creating compositions. *Experimenting* is Rubin's next stage. She named
it so because it is a time that the child is freely experimenting with all that
has incubated from previous stages and putting it together in their own style
of early representation. And *Consolidating* is the stage in which it all comes

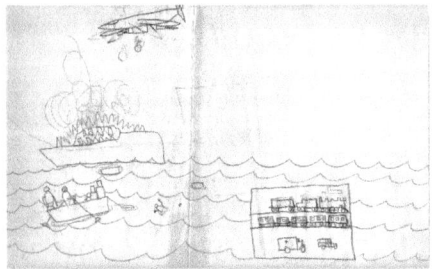

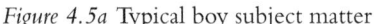

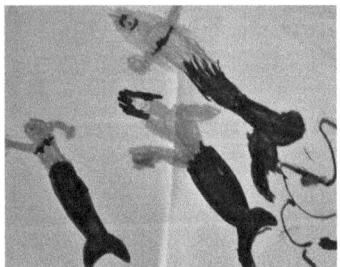

Figure 4.5a Typical boy subject matter   *Figure 4.5b* Typical girl subject matter

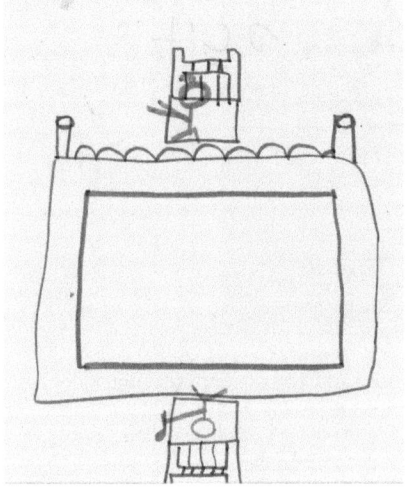

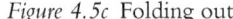

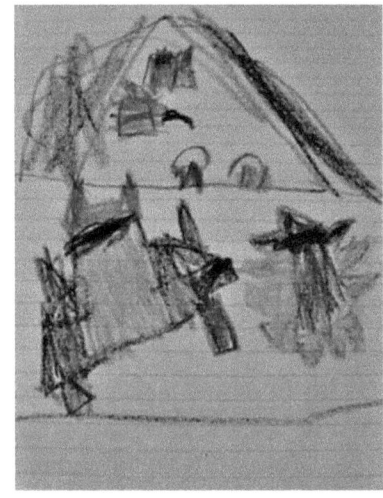

Figure 4.5c Folding out   *Figure 4.5d* Xray house

together in the child's art. Rubin relates it to their behavior which also becomes more organized and controlled as they move through school.

Gardner's stages for preschool and school-aged children are *Steps to a Doll House, Children's Drawings as Works of Art* (five to seven years) and *Reach Towards Realism* (eight to nine years). When Gardner discusses the stage called *Steps to a Doll House*, he follows the developmental progression of a young girl's art from scribbles, through forms, through human forms, through further addition of details to the ultimate end of the detailed doll house. He demonstrates how each step builds on the ones before to gel into this final representation.

Gardner makes a strong argument for *Children's Drawings as Works of Art.* He observes that so many facets of the child's personality are flowering as they enter school. They are singing, building more complexly with blocks, and telling stories. It stands to reason that their art would become more magnificent as they grow cognitively and socially/emotionally. As much as I appreciate the specifics of the three stages offered by Lowenfeld during the Latency Period, I agree with Gardner that children's drawings during these years are works of art.

My youngest son is a train enthusiast. From a young age, he laid track and created train layouts throughout the house. What was wonderful about his being so young with this endeavor was that he did not mind about scale, perspective, or proportion, in the way that an older child might. He just wanted to create this three-dimensional form from his own internal images and with what he had in the outside world. Different sizes of wooden trains,

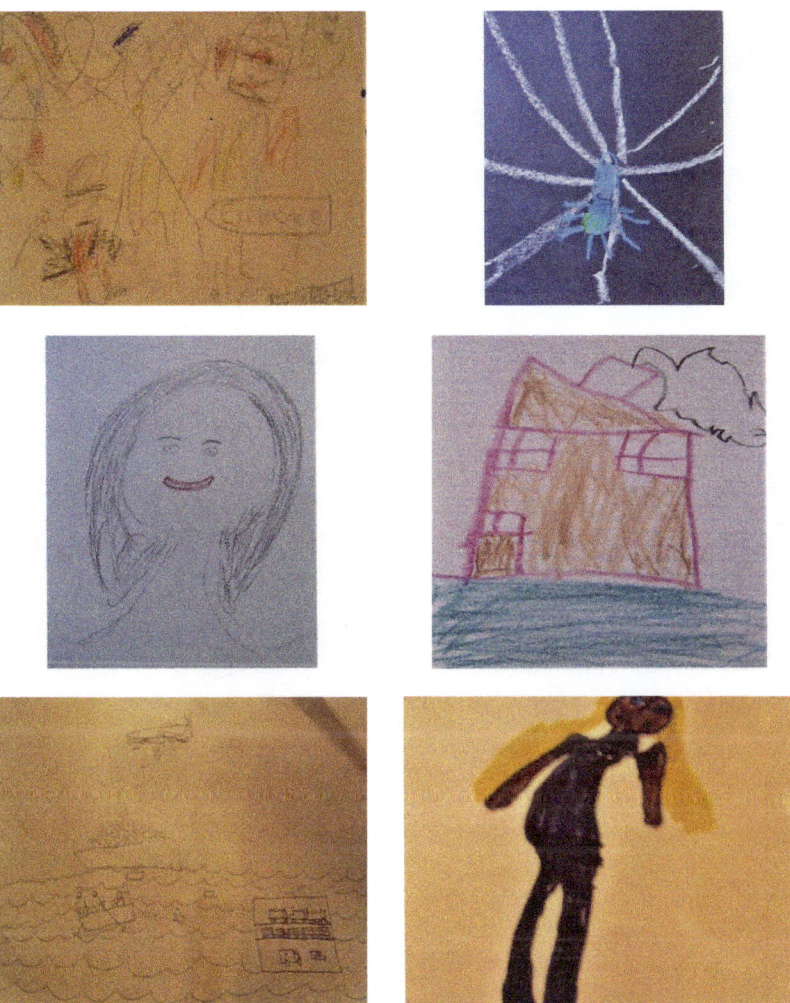

Chart 4.2 Typical latency period art

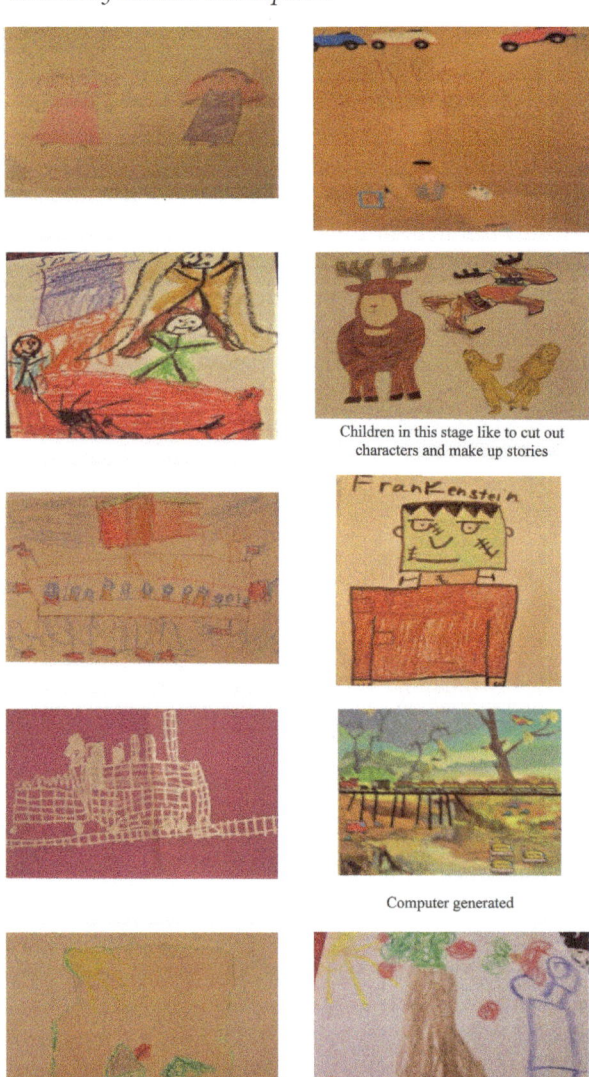

Children in this stage like to cut out
characters and make up stories

Computer generated

Chart 4.2 Continued

plastic trains, and all gauge of track were flanked by dollhouses, knickknack
houses and churches, Fisher Price® gas stations, parking garages, houses,
and barns. The town's population was whatever creatures accompanied the
structures. Cars and trucks were all brands and sizes, and wooden blocks,
plastic blocks, and brick blocks built the town. It was a magnificent work of
art, per Gardner.

Gardner bemoans the loss of this magic in his final stage of *Reach Towards Realism*. As the child is better able to represent perspective and proportion and present a more organized composition, he feels that their art is less aesthetic and expressive. Art becomes a bit more generic and less individual. Gardner does not like the loss of the magic and the slowly growing inhibition that occurs during this stage. In Figure 4.4, we see drawings about skateboarding by two brothers aged five and nine. The five-year old's drawing offers more of a magical experience. He is on his skateboard flying downhill with the word "COOL" in a bubble over his head. The nine-year old's drawing is less magical and more representational. He is carrying his skateboard, standing squarely on the groundline and more background detail is drawn.

Levick discusses her stages of *Sentence-Picture Stage/Sequence* (four to seven years) as the time when a child is speaking in full sentences and able to make themselves clear, and similarly, is developing more forms and organized composition in their art. During this stage, children are more influenced by and aware of their environment and culture. During the *Fact/Fantasy Stage/Sequence* (seven to 11 years), children are more aware of the difference between fact and fantasy and use their imaginations to learn more about themselves and their environment and express themselves with words and images.

DiLeo observes that at this stage, children's art is more dynamic in action and subject matter than the art of younger children. DiLeo refers to Luquet (1913) here explaining that when children draw, they demonstrate *Intellectual Realism* vs. *Visual Realism*. *Intellectual Realism* is defined as the child's attempt at representation and is from an internal model, being unconcerned with what the object looks like and reduces the schema to essentials, whereas

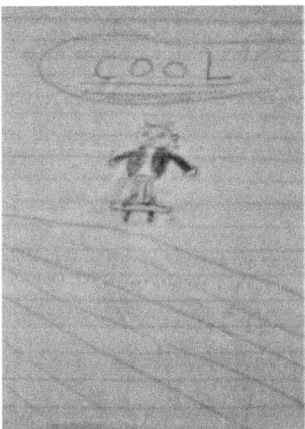 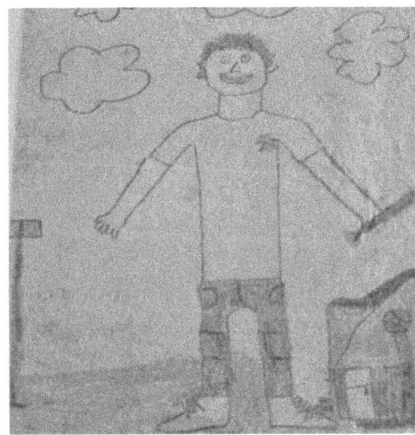

Figure 4.6 Comparison of *Children's Drawings as Works of Art* and *Reach Towards Realism*

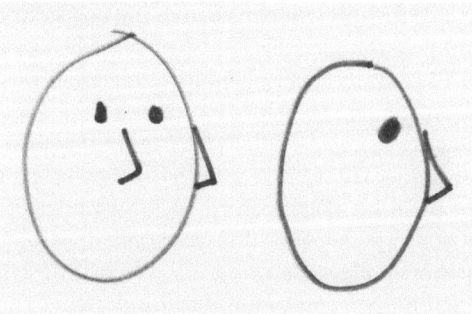

Figures 4.7 Author's rendering of mixed profile and correct profile orientation

Visual Realism is an adult's perception. As mentioned, DiLeo's stages are related to the development of the human form. During these years and as cognition matures, there are changes in the way the child represents human form. DiLeo identifies the early part of this phase as the *Transitional Stage* during which there is early or mixed profile representation and the later part of the phase brings *Correct Profile Orientation*.

Preschool Case

Charlie

Charlie was four years old when his mother brought him to me for art therapy. Charlie's Dad had taken him to Florida for two weeks per their custody agreement. While in Florida, Charlie stayed at his grandmother's house where his Dad lived, as well as Dad's 16-year-old brother. But he did not bring Charlie back at the end of the two weeks telling Charlie's Mom that he was going to keep him and pursue changes in their custody agreement. Charlie was there for four months. His father finally brought him back because he found out that his 16-year-old brother was sexually abusing Charlie, which added insult to injury. Charlie's Mom was understandably horrified and upset. When Charlie got home, his behavior was regressed. He was clinging to Mom and wetting the bed. Dad's brother admitted that there was touching and oral sex involved, but no penetration.

When Charlie came for art therapy, he wanted his Mom to stay in the room, and I agreed that was best for him. Charlie had been drawing human figures, but the art he did in his session was regressed. He approached the art with vehemence and represented oral dotting, anal denseness, and both urethral indulgent and aggressive lines creating art that looks like that of a younger child than he was.

In subsequent sessions, Charlie's art remained regressed. He smeared his drawing and drew penis-like projections and lots of heavy crossing out often found in the art of victims of sexual abuse. Charlie eventually seemed to move out of the anal stage into the urethral stage. He asked for watercolors and used excessive amounts of water. He applied the pigment and smeared the colors together until they were mostly brown. Charlie used so much water that we had to use paper towels to sop up some of the

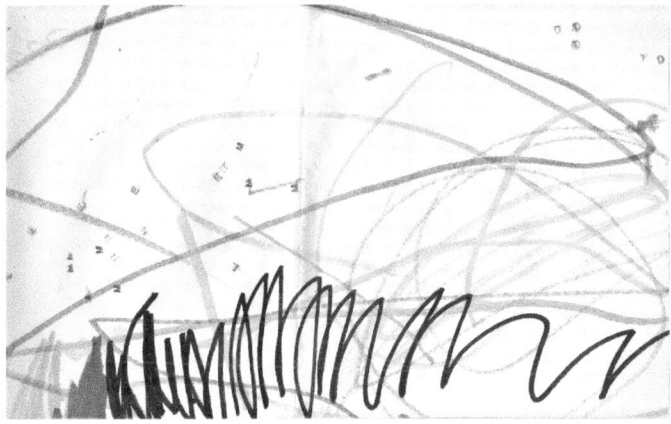

Figure 4.8a Charlie's first piece drawn with vehemence

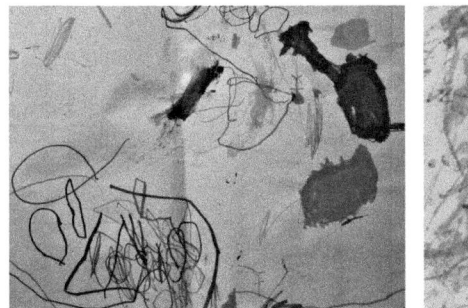 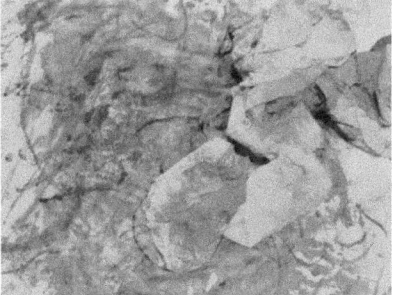

Figure 4.8b Charlie's anal art *Figure 4.8c* Charlie's urethral art

water. Charlie insisted on leaving the paper towels on the paper as part of the compos-ition, as if he were symbolically sopping up some of the fluids that were spilled by his uncle during the abuse. Charlie's bed wetting subsided after the urethral play, but he had many issues remaining to be solved.

School-aged Case

Doug

Doug was eight years old when his Mom brought him to me for art therapy. Doug was depressed and losing interest in everything. He wrote a story in school about wanting to die, and the school counselor strongly urged them to get him into therapy. His Mom informed me that his older brother had died in "an unfortunate accident" at the school the year before. Doug's Mom gave me no other information, and I suspected suicide. She dropped him off for his initial session with me and left to go shopping. I have

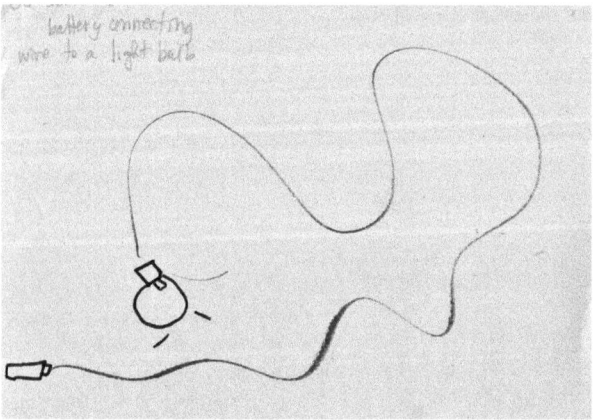

Figure 4.9 A wire with a lightbulb plugged into the wall

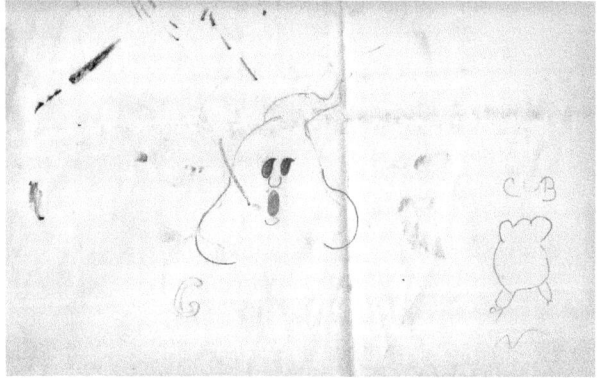

Figure 4.10 A ghost with something to say

to honestly say that was one of the most striking incidents I have experienced of a disconnected mother.

Doug did not want to be there and was very resistant to both making art and talking. I used the scribble technique (Winnicott, 1971b) with him, which I often use with kids to break the ice. Doug made very complicated scribbles, which were hard to make into anything. I purposely made simple scribbles to allow for more imagination on his part. During one session, Doug made my scribble into a wire with a lightbulb plugged into the wall. I understood this as his beginning to feel a connection to me so that he could gain some insight into what was going on in his life. After that session, Doug drew and spoke more freely.

Apparently, no one in his family, his mother, father, and three sisters, spoke about his late brother and how he had died, nor did anyone answer his questions. This was particularly difficult for Doug because, being the only other boy in the family, extended family members, teachers, and coaches were constantly comparing him to his brother saying things like he looked just like him, played soccer just like him, and so on. Doug never talked about his brother, but his symbolism was related. Doug was obsessed with the movie Ghostbusters *and often drew the logo. He also drew ghost images often, many of them had oral dotting indicating issues with attachment and separation. It is no wonder because no one at home was attached to anyone else, and no one discussed the ghost among them.*

Doug came in one day and was very angry. He told me it was his last session. I tried to convince his mother otherwise, but she was unmovable. I suppose Doug's wanting to talk more about the ghost in the family was too much for her.

Preadolescence and Adolescence

Freud labeled the preadolescent and adolescent years, which include the onset of puberty, the *Genital Stage.* This is the point in human development when sexual urges awaken through hormonal changes and which marks the beginning of adult sexuality. Piaget identifies this stage as *Formal Operations,* which marks the stage at which there is cognitive maturity for abstract and higher thinking and reasoning. During this stage, adolescents have a clearer and more integrated sense of morality, mores, and cultural expectations. This stage in Erikson's psychosocial model is *Identity vs. Role Confusion.* During these years adolescents learn more about themselves and develop belief systems. They begin to make plans for the future and think about college and careers. Relationships become important—both friendships and early intimate relationships.

Lowenfeld and Rubin are two developmental art theorists who describe and discuss these years. Lowenfeld delineates two phases in adolescence: *Age of Reason* and *Age of Decision.* He discusses the early part of this stage, the *Age of Reason,* as the true point in development where adolescents are capable of understanding abstractions and think reasonably. Because of this maturing cognition, adolescents now have a sense of perspective and proportion. Seventh grade art curricula usually include drawing the vanishing point with a pencil and a ruler. A younger child would have difficulty with this because their brains have not yet developed this capacity. Lowenfeld discusses the latter part of this phase, the *Age of Decision,* as a time for adolescents to experiment with a variety of media and engage in technical arts. Such use of art processes can enhance an academic curriculum, as well as offer adolescents an opportunity to explore career paths.

Rubin's two sequential phases that span the preadolescent and adolescent years are *Naturalizing* and *Personalizing /Aestheticizing.* During the *Naturalizing* stage, the preadolescent still has some of the adventurous attitude of latency years, and so, their art becomes more naturalistic. There is an increase in details overall with a more sophisticated awareness of spatial reality. Drawings of human forms include more details and a gradual sense of body parts in proportion to the rest of the body and to the environment.

Rubin points out that it is during the transition from the *Naturalizing* stage to the *Personalizing /Aestheticizing* stage that many children become discouraged with their art ability and will leave artmaking behind. However, she also feels that supportive art training would certainly help some of these discouraged young artists to hang on. The *Personalizing /Aestheticizing* stage includes older adolescents. At this point, they are comfortable with their art ability and strive to make their art representative of who they are, or who they are becoming. They want to personally represent and express their perception of their world within and without and do so aesthetically. The adolescent is consciously in charge of their art, whether working in a free or controlled manner.

Preadolescence

Defining preadolescence as separate from adolescence is useful for effective treatment. They are distinct in many ways but also alike. Some preadolescents go through puberty before the teenage years. Others do not and still look like elementary aged children, but hormones are percolating. Almost every preadolescent cannot wait to become a teenager. The world around them expects maturity but encourages them to enjoy being kids. There is need for concern here because preadolescents' grasp of abstract concepts is not fully developed and may interfere with their judgment, such as engaging in risky behaviors with peers because they do not have a full sense of consequences.

For quite a while, *tween* has been used colloquially to identify this age group. However, I get the distinct feeling from my patients of this age and my sisters' grandchildren that this is not a preferential term. Personally, I think it is a perfect term because preadolescents are right in between being children and being teenagers. However, I do not wish to be politically incorrect and I do wish to be respectful, so I will use preadolescent as an identifying term.

Early adolescence is the time in life when many people stop making art. It is a tumultuous time in development for everyone. If one is not skillful at drawing, while suffering the many insecurities of this age, one will stop drawing. The example I offer to students is to imagine that the girl sitting next to you is drawing a beautiful horse that looks like Black Beauty, and your rendering of a horse looks like a rectangle with stick legs coming out. You most likely will stop drawing to protect your ego from further insults.

Preadolescence is a hard time in development, and consequently, a hard age group with whom to do treatment. When I meet with a preadolescent for an initial session, I ask them if they want their parents to come into the session. Younger children usually assume their parents will join in the initial session, and adolescents usually assume their parents will not come into the initial session. By giving them the choice, I am allowing them to tell me which option is more comfortable for them.

Allowing preadolescents, the opportunity to express their feelings in art is important because they have so many confusing feelings. Getting these feelings,

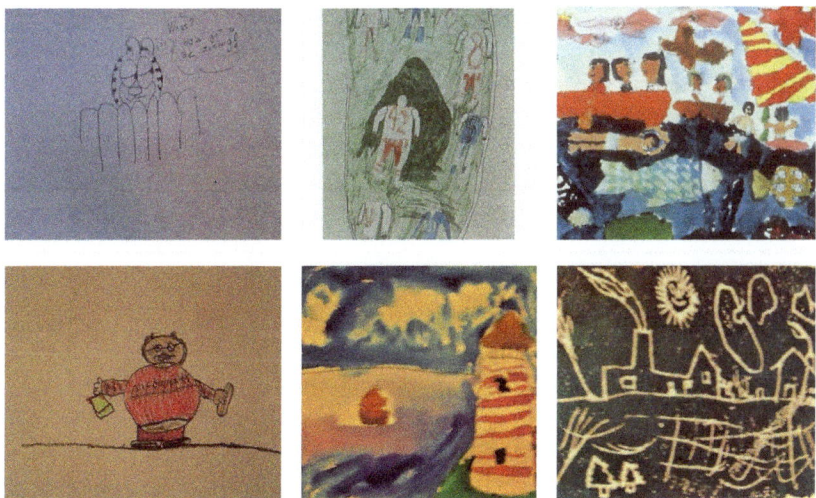

Chart 4.3 Typical preadolescent art

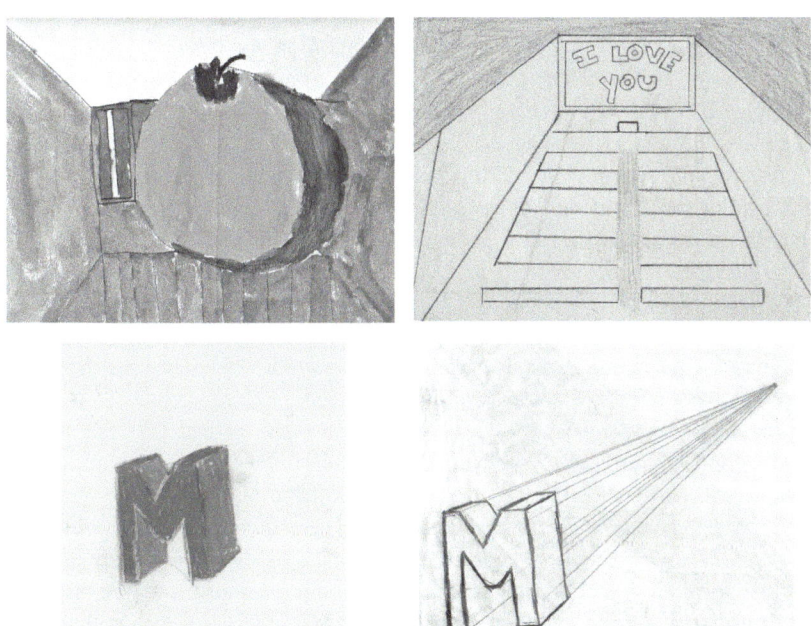

Figures 4.11a, b, c, and d Exercises in perspective

emotions, and issues out in an artform allows them to look at them more objectively and process them with a creative arts therapist. Acknowledging that preadolescents may not be comfortable with drawing, it is important to offer other options for expression, like photography or collage.

Young adolescents like to practice drawing with perspective which is something they are learning to do and further are understanding developmentally. With this newly acquired skill, they can use rulers and pencils with erasers and change their minds or correct errors.

Preadolescent Case

Harry

Harry was 11 years old when his parents brought him to art therapy. They were concerned that he was very depressed. They came into the initial session with him because he refused to talk. Harry's Mom had filled me in on significant history via a phone call. When Harry was 11 months old, his sister was born, and due to birth complications, she had severe cerebral palsy and was very debilitated. From that point in Harry's life and until he was almost three years old, he was primarily in the care of his grandparents, while his parents took care of his sister. She was often hospitalized and had many regular appointments with specialists. Now, when Harry was 11 years old, his parents were beginning to pursue legal channels to sue for malpractice to secure funding for his sister's constant needs and care. This triggered Harry's deep-seated sense of abandonment and he became significantly depressed. I assured his Mom that she was making the right decision getting him into therapy because depression can be deadly and must be taken seriously.

In the initial session with his parents and for a few sessions afterwards, Harry sat in silence with his sweatshirt zipped up and the hood pulled tightly around his face. I explained to his Mom, at that point, that I was allowing him the silence because he would talk when he was ready and felt he could trust me. His parents trusted my professional judgment and understood.

Near the end of the third session of silence and avoidance, I said, "You know, Harry, you can say a lot without words." Tears began to trickle down his cheek. He dried them and left the session without saying a word.

The next week, Harry came in and wanted to make art and talk. He made a cartoon-like clay creature who lived on Mars. He called him Li'l HH, which were his initials, and he was 11 months old. Harry explained to me that creatures on Mars could express themselves in words and make their needs known by 11 months. How poignant. Harry was unable to do this and so gave the ability to do so to his alter ego. He worked on drawings of creatures and scenery in this alternative universe for several weeks. Harry introduced other characters and places. I could not make any interpretations because it would have scared Harry off. Rather, I worked with the metaphor and marveled at how Li'l HH was so lucky that he could tell people what he needed and how he felt. Li'l HH was also lucky because he had a good support system— all the other characters introduced took care of or were great friends with Li'l HH. Harry's rendering of Li'l HH's planet shows a world that hovers with no base, and he explained that the occupants of Li'l HH's planet are able to negotiate this. I thought

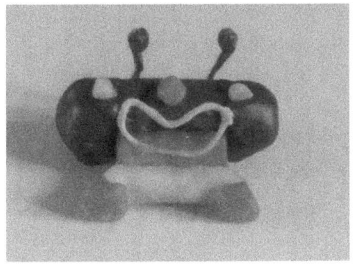
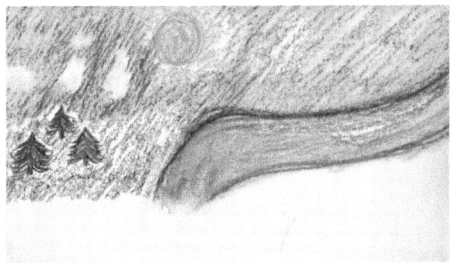

Figure 4.12a Li'l HH   *Figure 4.12b Li'l HH's home planet*

that maybe Harry was telling me that he was beginning to negotiate his world that had a missing base in his early development.

Harry got restless as things in his story got too close to his real life and wanted to leave therapy. His parents were wise and agreed with me that we needed a session together to terminate, or with any luck convince Harry to continue. I talked very frankly with Harry about depression and suicide, including referring to Kurt Cobain because Harry was a Nirvana fan.

"He was a drug addict. That's why he killed himself."

I explained to Harry that many people who suffer from depression self-medicate with drugs, but they do not all shoot themselves. I emphasized that depression is real, and rather than suffer, you can get help with therapy or even medication. I urged him to listen to what I was saying and made him promise his parents that he would ask for help if he felt so bad that he wanted to hurt himself. Harry chose not to continue but got the idea of how to ask for and use therapy going forward in his life.

Adolescence

Anna Freud (1969) calls adolescence a normal developmental disturbance:

> …it has struck me always as unfortunate that the period of adolescent upheaval and inner arrangement of forces coincides with such major demands on the individual as those for academic achievements in school and college, for a choice of career, for increased social and financial responsibility in general. Many failures, often with tragic consequences in these respects, are not due to the individual's incapacity as such but more to the fact that such demands are made on him at a time of life when all energies are engaged otherwise, namely, in trying to solve the major problems created for him by normal sexual growth and development.
>
> (p. 10)

There is little more for me to say about adolescence than Freud said here. The transition to adulthood is, perhaps, the most significant one in anyone's life. Everything that has happened in development up to that point is now pushing through this transition. If someone has had healthy psychosexual, cognitive, and psychosocial development, the outcomes will be better with a prognosis for a fulfilling adult life. If not, there will be more obstacles to overcome with poorer resources. Either way, it is not easy.

When I was teaching classes on developmental art therapy, it occurred to me that the artwork of adolescents, which I was showing to students in class, was from adolescents who could be identified as having disturbances. They had cognitive, behavioral, and emotional issues. I decided that to be fair to both my students and other typically developing adolescents, I wanted to gather and show artwork of the latter. To my surprise, at first, the artwork given to me by typically developing adolescents was not so different from the artwork I had from adolescents with difficulties. On further reflection, I realized that this was, of course, the case because all adolescents are dealing with upheaval during these years of life.

It is a time of turmoil and a search for identity. The transition here is from childhood into adolescence, and the separation/individuation during these years is both from those childhood years and the family in which those attachments are formed. Adolescents reflect on their childhood and make decisions, both consciously and unconsciously, about what they want and need to keep and assimilate and what they want and need to move away from as they move forward—often what they want to eliminate are those attachments to their parents. Adolescents want to form a self-identity. Being rebellious is part of being an adolescent, and of course, rejecting or revising the beliefs and values of their parents is part of their growth towards self-identity.

When I did an intake interview with a 15-year-old girl on an inpatient behavioral health unit, I got a snapshot of this path on her journey. Lindsay had slashed her wrists the night before in a suicide attempt. Before I sat down with her, I reviewed her chart. She had a history of serious acting out and self-harm. Her parents were both physicians in the hospital, and I felt that part of her motivation in hurting herself was to embarrass them. After I asked her the usual questions and asked if she could contract for safety, I encouraged Lindsay to tell me more about herself and her friends. She went into great detail about the fact that she was a Wiccan in her belief system and rejected her parents' religion. Life is very sacred in Wicca, she informed me. Lindsay stated to me, with conviction, that followers of Wicca believe that if you cause harm to something, it comes back to you many-fold. I pointed to her stitched and bandaged wrists and asked her how one would defend that as a Wiccan. Lindsay glared at me with anger in her eyes and said, "Well, I've only been Wiccan since Tuesday!!" In other words, adult person, stop challenging my beliefs! I often tell this story because I think it epitomizes the fluid nature of the adolescent ego as it pushes and pulls towards self-identity.

When working with adolescents, it is important to treat them with respect, acknowledging that they are going through a hard time. Being supportive will engender trust, which will enable them to share what is on their mind and why. The matter of trust emerges immediately when working with adolescents when it comes to the issues of confidentiality.

I will assure them that what they tell me or draw stays in the session unless I am concerned that they are going to hurt themselves or someone else. Then, I will tell their parents (or school staff or hospital staff) and will do so with them present if they so choose. Regarding the subject matter of the art, adolescents will often draw provocative images. Again, I inform them that I will not censor or judge what they draw but will engage in conversation on the topic with them. Regarding their clothing, however, in a school or hospital setting, there were restrictions on what they could wear and were not allowed to wear anything that had gang symbols, images of violence, inappropriate sexual imagery, Satanic references, and drug or alcohol imagery. Such imagery is inappropriate if people are detoxing and upsetting if people are actively psychotic.

The idea of censorship can be a powder keg with adolescents. Haeseler (1987) discusses this topic thoroughly regarding a situation with adolescents on an inpatient behavioral health unit. In a group, adolescents expressed their anger at the administration in a mural using violent and offensive imagery, feeling they were told they could draw whatever they wanted to. While this angry mural was fine within the confines of the group space, displaying it on a unit that also housed patients with psychosis or anxiety was inappropriate. This had to be processed and explained to the kids, but the fine line between trust and mistrust can easily be breached with adolescents.

Working as an art therapist in a special education junior and senior high school was a challenge. Gaining trust was essential. I felt strongly that treating the kids as if they were typical pre-teens and teens would provide a healing environment, and it proved to be beneficial. For part of their English Language Arts curriculum, the students published their own school paper, including their poems, essays, and editorials. This expanded to a yearbook in which they included the photography that they used for their Fine Arts curriculum. The students had a full photography and ceramics studio with teaching artists who worked with them. I scoured the country until I found a do-it-yourself yearbook company through which we could publish the 60 or so yearbooks that we needed for this small school. I also scoured NYC looking for a jeweler who would make the 12 class rings for our graduates, as opposed to the usual order of hundreds from public schools. We had a prom for the entire school. We decorated the common room like a tropical paradise. One of the art therapists had gone to a large public high school in the suburbs and attended a few proms and was then in several of her friends' bridal parties. She generously brought in nearly a dozen formal gowns for the girls to choose from and keep. We also recruited other staff members to dress the boys, do hair and make-up for anyone that wanted it, and lend jewelry. There was a photo station for souvenir pictures. They could have as many pictures taken as they wanted with all combinations of friends, and the photo staff printed out the pictures (in the darkroom—no digital photography then!) for the kids during the next week of school at no charge. We had a grant from Polaroid® and used their cameras and film throughout the school year and across the curriculum. But, at the prom, there were cameras for them to take casual shots of each other, which we posted on the common bulletin board. I am not sure, but I think we had more fun than the kids did, but it was fun all around. The results of treating the kids like they were in a "normal" school paid off. No one acted out at the prom, and they were all clean and sober, as best as we could tell. Attendance and academic perform-ance improved, and pre-test and post-test research that we were conducting indicated improvement in self-esteem and personal responsibility.

Adolescents love to do graffiti. It usually includes their *Tag* name, or nickname. It supports self-identity, and being stylized, it allows for easier self-expression, per Lowenfeld's *Age of Decision* and Rubin's *Aestheticizing*. Similarly, words often appear along with drawings, also making a personal statement.

Adolescents often draw mosaic patterns and fill them in. Of course, this requires minimal art ability, so it is a good way to express themselves. I started to notice that they often left some of the spaces uncolored. At first, I thought this was indicative of an issue, but then I noticed that the kids that were doing well did this. I hypothesized that this was their way of filling in important things in their lives and leaving room for growth.

Satanic or occult symbols appear often because they are experimenting and trying to find something they can believe in or relate to. Adolescents

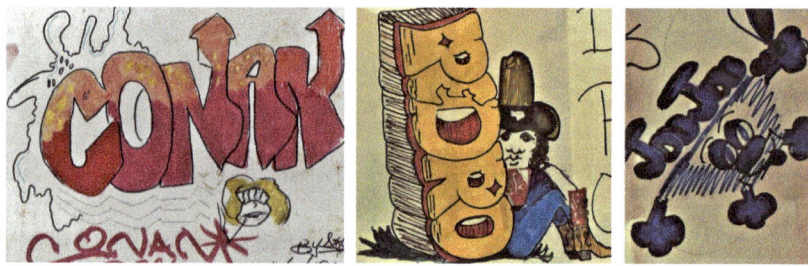

Figures 4.13 Graffiti

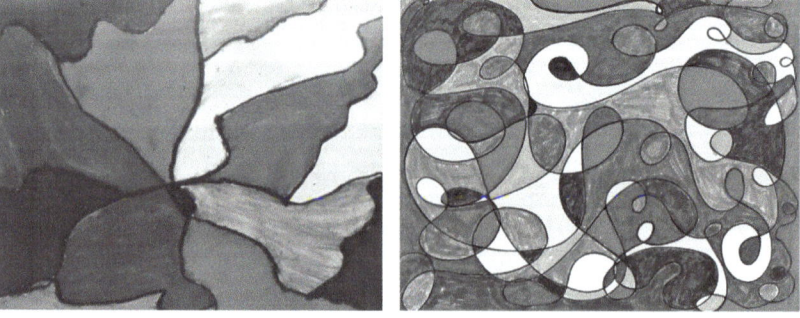

Figures 4.14 Mosaics with uncolored spaces

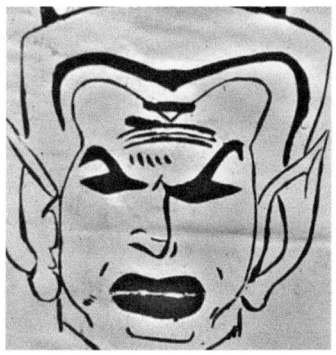 

Figures 4.15 Provocative subject matter

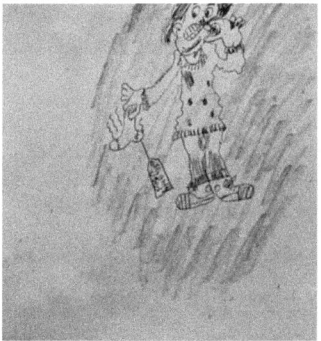 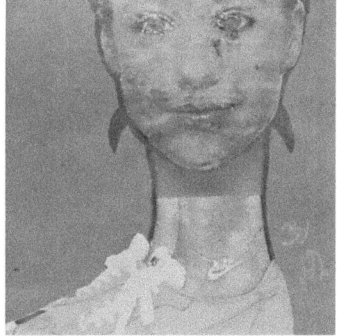

Figures 4.16 Cartoon characters

often draw other provocative subject matter because being oppositional and provocative is part of being an adolescent.

Adolescents draw cartoon figures. Often, these are of their own creation and become their characters who have adventures and stories that go with them.

Below is adolescent art created by both typical teens and atypical teens. In fact, some of it was done by adults with addictions and mental illness, who often draw at an adolescent level, including subject matter and execution. Addictions counselors say that a person's development stops at the age that they start using. Per Anna Freud's (1969) acknowledgment that adolescence is a developmental disturbance, differences between and among are insignificant.

Adolescent Case

Aisha

Aisha was a 15-year-old girl, who did art therapy with me in a special education school. Aisha had some behavioral problems and learning difficulties but was open to

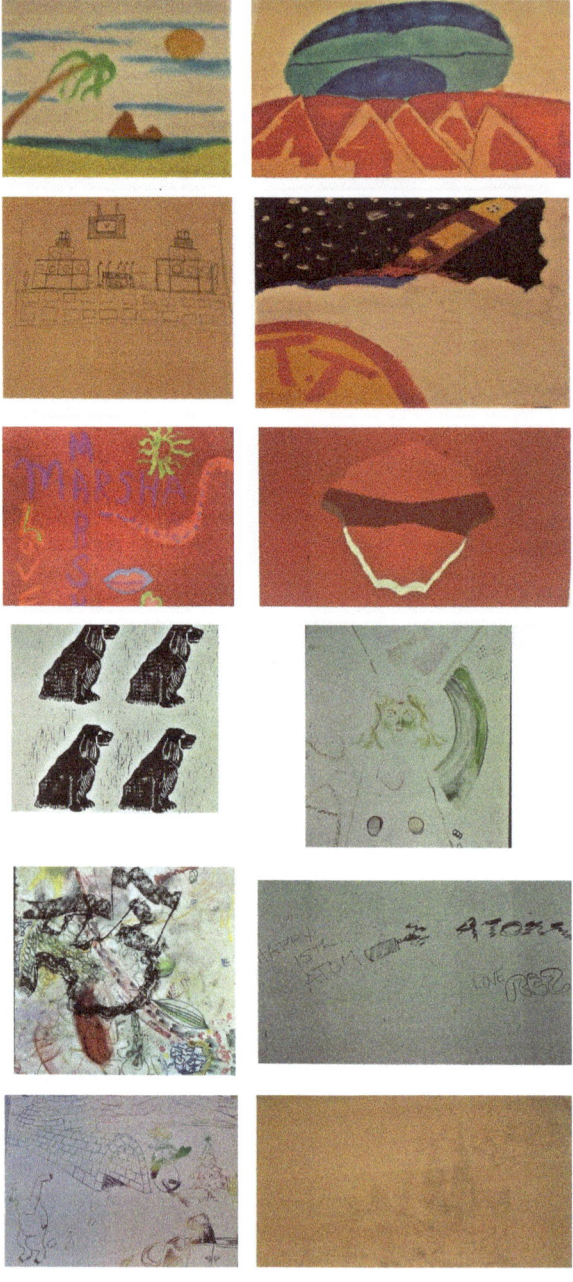

Chart 4.4 Adolescent Art

learning about herself in therapy. She always came on time and engaged easily. At first, Aisha kept things superficial, but as time went on, she shared more about her dysfunctional home life. Aisha's older sister prostituted for drugs and was rarely around. Aisha's mother was a serious alcoholic. She did not work and drank most of the day, when she was awake, and then went out to bars at night. Aisha explained to me that she usually came home to an empty house, made her own dinner, and tried to do her homework without support. If she woke up, and her mother was not home, Aisha went out looking for her, brought her home, and put her to bed. Consequently, Aisha was often tired and preoccupied during the school day. In this picture, though Aisha said it was a man, I think she is representing her home life. The man is the only one on an empty island. He is fishing which may represent Aisha's nightly task of trying to find her mother and reel her in. The tree, drawn with light oral indulgent lines, leans heavily on the man and may represent Aisha's burden. Three coconuts are the strongest image in that tree and appear to be looking down on her. Maybe they represent those of us who tried to look over her.

One day, Aisha came into the art room and told me she was tired. She put her head down on my desk and was immediately asleep. Because we had been dealing with heavy issues, I first thought she may have been resistant to having a session that day. But then I looked at her and saw that she was sleeping very deeply and peacefully. I let her sleep and woke her up gently so that she would be on time for her next class. Aisha stretched, got up, hugged me, and said, "Thank you, Miss Beth." I realized that I had provided her with a safe holding environment where she could rest well and not have to worry about things that she should not have to worry about. One of the last pieces of art that Aisha made in art therapy, which she gave to me, was a house. While this looks like a typical adolescent rendering of a house, on inspection, there is no door to enter or exit, some of the windows are X'ed out possibly meaning taboo, and dark smoke comes from the chimney, which can indicate stress in the home. It is also a country home and not the apartment in the projects where she lived. I think it was Aisha's way of letting me know that the holding environment which I had provided her helped her negotiate her dysfunctional home.

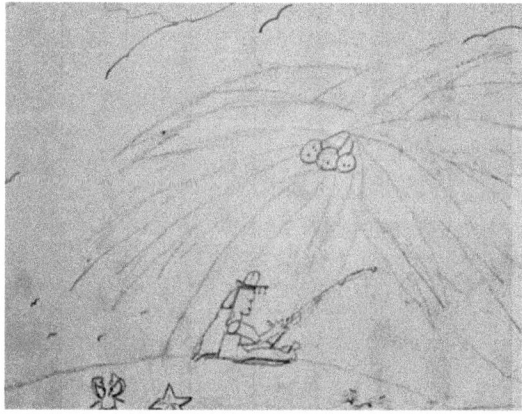

Figure 4.17 Aisha's island

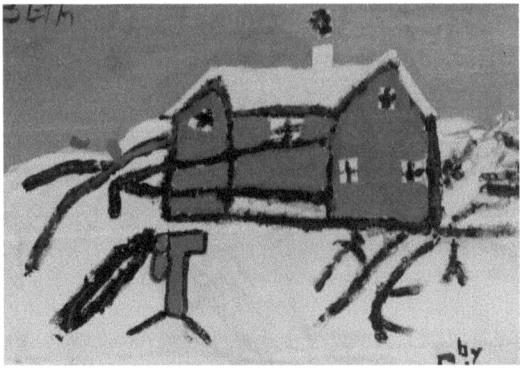

Figure 4.18 Aisha's house

Adulthood

Piaget (1973) offers a suggestion of a distinct stage that represents development during the ages from 15 to 20 years of age. He remarks that this stage is more dependent on innate ability and societal demands than simply cognition. The research presented and discussed by Piaget investigates his stages of cognitive development. He hypothesizes that his delineated stages of development will occur sequentially with some expected variation regarding age and ability. However, in the research quoted, the older adolescents/young adult group demonstrated a great diversification in abilities. While all mature to the point of being able to develop formal structure, there is a great difference in their application of this cognitive growth. All typically developing children maturing in the stage of concrete operations will approach, understand, and execute a task similarly. However, some young adults may be able to do the same with a physics problem, and others will not; but those others are able to engage in art or literary work with the ease that the original some cannot. Piaget concludes that this can, therefore, not be characterized as a proper stage of cognitive development towards adulthood, but rather a "structural advancement in the direction of specialization" (p. 208).

Erikson was one of the first developmental theorists to offer developmental stages that span the life cycle, seeing adulthood as another stage. In his psychosocial model, Erikson breaks adulthood into three stages: Early adulthood is identified as the stage of *Intimacy vs. Isolation*; middle adulthood as *Generativity vs. Stagnation*; and the older years as *Ego Integrity vs. Despair*.

During *Intimacy vs. Isolation*, young adults often become involved in long-term intimate relationships. It is also a time in life when one embarks on a job or career path, which can offer a sense of intimacy with people of similar goals or interests. Erikson describes the middle years as *Generativity vs. Stagnation*. It is during this time, that most adults are in a job or career for several years and becoming more of a master in their trade. Simultaneously, adults in this stage may be having or growing families and become more active and productive in their communities. Erikson describes the older years, the stage of *Ego Integrity vs. Despair*, as a time when one reviews what they have accomplished in their life to the end of feeling a sense of personal integrity.

A nurse gerontologist, Naomi Feil (1973) added a stage in the spirit of Erikson entitled *Validation vs. Vegetation*. Feil's work was predominantly with patients suffering with dementia. She suggests that some of the confusion and dementia may be the person's way of blocking out painful life experiences or warding off despair. Her research indicates that validating the person's confusion rather than dismissing it can create better communication between that person and their caregiver.

The theorists of art development have not identified stages of adult art. If adults have artistic aptitude or abilities, they may engage in art as a profession or a vocation. Interestingly, sometimes the art of these adults is stylized to the point of presenting as resistance in art therapy. As mentioned, most adults stop making art when they are 11 or 12 years of age if it is not something, they are good at. And for the most part, they will not easily engage in art during art therapy stating, "I have not drawn since 7th grade" or "This is for kids" or "I should give these markers to my grandkids—they'll do better than me."

When I review the art of adults, I use a developmental model to better understand their issues and when they may have occurred and how the pattern keeps repeating.

Adulthood Case

Gene

Gene was 28 when he entered art therapy with me. Gene was just one of those people that never finished anything he started. He left college seven years earlier needing only six credits for his B.A. He would cut off any intimate relationships when they were going somewhere, and he never stayed long at a job. Gene did have some good long-term friends, but he saw them moving forward with their lives, and he was not. It was clear to me that Gene did not want to be successful. In his family, that was not always a good thing. His father ran a successful business, but Gene knew his father was a womanizer because he had the misfortune to be home from school when his father brought a woman home. His mother was a successful executive secretary but really did not care about much else and was cold towards everyone, including Gene, the baby of six. His older brother was a successful attorney and a lay deacon in their Church, but he was a closeted gay man and led a secret life. His four sisters were successful and had no secret lives that mattered in therapy, but they all babied Gene and had done so his entire life. They even called him "Baby." It is easy to see that Gene had secondary

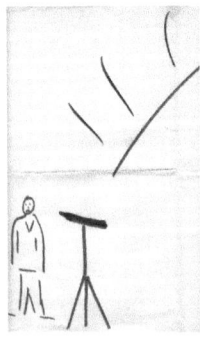

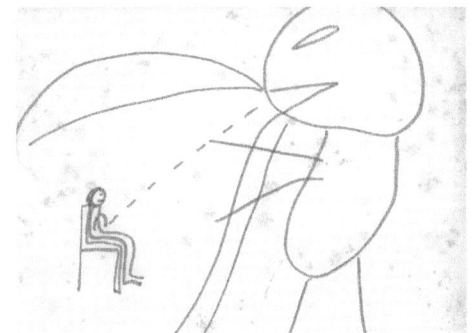

Figure 4.19a Gene over whelmed

Figure 4.19b Gene being scolded by his brother

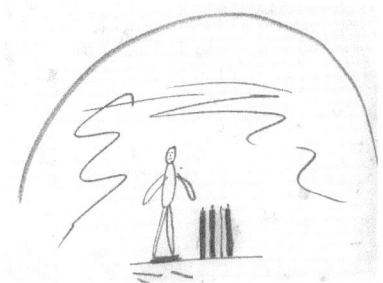

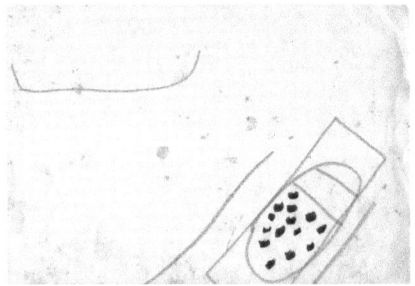

Figure 4.19c Gene on the side of the road

Figure 4.19d "You have too much baggage!"

gains in remaining a failure, but he knew things had to change. Gene had no role models to show him what it is like to be a balanced and responsible adult.

Gene drew himself trying to look forward (Figure 4.19a). His self-representations were always made up of disconnected light lines, oral indulgent. Gene seems to have no self-image, and he can see no one through the telescope reflecting back to him. Rather there is an overarching sun, which most likely represents his father. There was rarely a groundline in his art, which appears in the Pre-schematic Stage. Developmentally, Gene is about five years old in many ways. Figure 4.19b is Gene's brother lecturing him, with oral dotting and urethral indulgent lines spewing onto him from his brother's mouth. My sense is that this represents Gene's ambivalence between staying attached and running away. Figures 4.19c and dare a dream that Gene reported. He was on his way to meet his friends at a weekend resort, and his car broke down. He can see the resort from where he broke down. Gene is standing there with his suitcases. He does have a groundline and more of a sense of self as

DLIEO	GARDNER	KELLOGG	KESTENBERG	LEVICK	LOWENFELD	RUBIN
UNRECOGNIZABLE REPRESENTATIONS	SCRUBBLING— BABBLING	BASIC SCRIBBLES (under 2)	ORAL (0–10 months)	BABBLE-SCRIBBLE STAGE/SEQUENCE (18 mos.–2-1/2 yrs.)	SCRUBBLING: (2–4 years)	MANIPULATING
	ROMANCE WITH FORMS	PLACEMENT PATTERNS (2–4 years)	ANAL (10–20 months)		1. disordered	FORMING
	1. patterners 2. dramatists			WORD-SHAPE STAGE/SEQUENCE (2–1/2 to 4 years)	2. controlled 3. named	NAMING
TADPOLE STAGE	TADPOLES	TWO SHAPE STAGE (3–4 years) 1. implied 2. outline	URETHRAL (20–30 months)	SENTENCE-PICTURE STAGE/SEQUENCE (4–7 years)	PRE-SCHEMATIC (4–7 years)	REPRESENTING
TRANSITIONAL STAGE (trunk appears)	TRANSITIONAL STAGE AS THINGS.	DESIGN STAGE (3–5 years)	INNER GENITAL (30–48 months)			CONTAINING
FULL FACE WITH PROGRESSIVE ADDITION OF BODY PARTS	STEPS TO A DOLL HOUSE	EARLY PICTORIAL STAGE (5 years)	OUTER GENITAL (48–60 months)			EXPERIMENTING
TRANSITIONAL STAGE (early profile representation)	CHILDREN'S DRAWINGS AS WORKS OF ART (5–7 years)	LATER PICTORIAL STAGE (5–7 yrs.)		FACT-FANTASY STAGE/SEQUENCE (7–11 years)	SCHEMATIC (7–9 years)	CONSOLIDATING
CORRECT PROFILE ORIENTATION	REACH TOWARDS REALISM (8–9 years)	FINAL STAGE (7 on) self taught art			DAWNING REALISM (9–12 years)	NATURALIZING
					PSEUDO-NATURALISM (adolescence)	PERSONALIZING /
					1. Age of Reason 2. Age of Decision	AESTHETICIZING

Chart 4.5 Developmental art Theorists

urethral aggressive signature lines float above his head. Along comes a big convertible Cadillac with all of his friends inside. When he asks if they can give him a ride, they all say, "No. Sorry. You have too much baggage." And they drove away. It took a while, but Gene began to understand this dream. But true to form, as Gene got closer to working on his issues, he left therapy.

5   Trauma

In 1996, Shirley Riley was predicting what near future needs would be in art therapy treatment which, therefore, should be addressed in art therapy education. She felt that art therapists needed to educate themselves more regarding legal matters, changing families, addictions, and trauma.

And she was right, specifically by highlighting trauma. Increasing interaction with the legal system, changing families, and addictions all indicate trauma, personal and societal. In 2003, I (Gonzalez-Dolginko, 2003) wrote a brief report stating that art therapists need to prepare themselves for dealing with trauma because it is here to stay. Many clinicians began to realize that trauma was not just something that happens here and there. It happens everywhere and to everyone. There are few patients we treat who are not dealing with trauma in some way from their lived experience. I can honestly say that in my 46 years of practice, every patient I treated suffered trauma. This trauma could be horrific abuse or the loss of a beloved grandparent, but it is trauma and leaves a mark on a person's heart and soul. This is the history a patient brings into the session, and considering when this trauma occurred during their development offers insight into how to proceed in treatment.

The last half of the 20th Century became increasingly traumatic for the world at large— the Cold War, terrorism, famine, nuclear disasters, natural disasters, AIDS and other epidemics and pandemics, despotic rulers, climate change. And these have continued into the 21st Century. Creative arts therapists must mitigate their own trauma while treating patients for trauma and be careful of vicarious traumatization (Baird & Kracen, 2006). Van der Kolk, McFarlane, and Weisaeth (1996) discuss trauma as a human condition and what pushes evolution forward, but the stress caused by trauma can be overwhelming on the mind, body, and society.

Much of the world's population is experiencing cumulative trauma, which adds another degree of difficulty onto the treatment process. Cumulative trauma is relatively undocumented in art therapy practice, although there is growing evidence that art therapy provides distinct benefits for resolving various traumas. Naff (2014) proposes an art therapy treatment framework for cumulative trauma derived from semi-structured interviews with art therapists and artistic representations of their approaches. In art therapy treatment, Naff advises attention to the variability of symptom presentation, a clear treatment approach, and the use of art as a treatment modality to support nonverbal expression.

Psychological trauma is an affliction of the powerless. At the moment that the trauma occurs, the victim is rendered helpless by overwhelming force. When the force is that of nature, we speak of disasters. When the force is that of other human beings, we speak of atrocities. Traumatic events overwhelm the ordinary systems of care that give people a sense of control, connection, and meaning.

Posttraumatic Stress Disorder, or PTSD, is a psychiatric disorder that can occur following the experience or witnessing of life-threatening events such as military combat, natural disasters, terrorist incidents, serious accidents, or violent personal assaults, like rape. People who suffer from PTSD often relive the experience through nightmares and flashbacks, have difficulty sleeping, and feel detached or estranged, and these symptoms can be severe enough and last long enough to significantly impair the person's daily life.

PTSD is not a new disorder. There are written accounts of similar symptoms that go back to ancient times, and there is clear documentation in the historical medical literature starting with the Civil War. There are particularly good descriptions of posttraumatic stress symptoms in the medical literature on combat veterans of World War II and on Holocaust survivors. Careful research and documentation of PTSD began in earnest after the Vietnam War. In 1988, reports indicate that 15.2% of Vietnam vets were suffering from it and that 30% had experienced the disorder at some point since returning from Vietnam. PTSD has subsequently been observed in all veteran populations that have been studied, including World War II, Korean conflict, and Persian Gulf populations, and in United Nations peace-keeping forces deployed to other war zones around the world (Rothbaum et al., 2000).

PTSD is not only a problem for veterans. While there are unique cultural- and gender-based aspects of the disorder, it occurs in men and women, adults and children, Western and non-Western cultural groups, and all socio-economic strata. Most people who are exposed to a traumatic, stressful event experience some of the symptoms of PTSD in the days and weeks following exposure. Data suggest that about 8% of men and 20% of women go on to develop PTSD, and roughly 30% of these individuals develop a chronic form that persists throughout their lifetimes (Rothbaum et al., 2000).

Chronic PTSD usually involves periods of symptom increase followed by remission or decrease, although some individuals may experience symptoms that are unremitting and severe. Some older veterans, for example, who report a lifetime of only mild symptoms, experience significant increases in symptoms following retirement. Other triggers may be severe medical illness in themselves or their spouses and reminders of their military service, such as reunions or media broadcasts of the anniversaries of war events.

PTSD (Rothbaum et al., 2000) is marked by clear biological changes as well as psychological symptoms. Other problems of physical and mental health include impairment of the person's ability to function in social or family life, occupational instability, marital problems and divorces, family discord, difficulties in parenting, and involvement with the criminal justice system.

Other symptoms of PTSD include: recurring thoughts or nightmares about the event; trouble sleeping and/or changes in appetite; increased anxiety, fear, and vigilance; overwhelming depression and low energy; memory lapses; feeling "scattered" or numb and unable to focus on work or daily activities; and an inability to face certain aspects of the trauma and avoidance of reminders of the event.

PTSD is associated with distinctive neurobiological and physiological changes (Rothschild, 2000). Psychophysiological alterations associated with PTSD include hyper-arousal of the sympathetic nervous system, increased sensitivity of the startle reflex, and sleep abnormalities. People with PTSD tend to have abnormal levels of key hormones involved in the body's response to stress. Thyroid function also seems to be enhanced in people with PTSD. Headaches, gastrointestinal complaints, immune system problems, dizziness, chest pain, and discomfort in other parts of the body are common in people with PTSD. Often, medical doctors treat the symptoms without being aware that they stem from PTSD.

People more sensitive to PTSD may experience greater stressor magnitude and intensity, unpredictability, uncontrollability, sexual (as opposed to non-sexual) victimization, real or perceived responsibility, and a sense of betrayal. Those with prior vulnerability factors such as genetics, early age of onset and longer-lasting childhood trauma, lack of functional social support, and concurrent stressful life events may experience PTSD more intensely. This is also true for those who report greater perceived threat or danger, suffering, upset, terror, and horror or fear, or are in a social environment that produces shame, guilt, stigmatization, or self-hatred. Ogden, Pain, and Fisher (2006) describe that traumatized individuals do not just suffer with memories of tragic and horrifying experiences; they demonstrate many complicated and debilitating signs, symptoms, and difficulties consisting primarily of bodily responses to dysregulated affects. These often have no clear subjective connection to their fragments of narrative memory.

PTSD is complicated by the fact that it frequently co-exists in conjunction with related disorders, such as depression, substance abuse, mood disorders, anxiety disorders, substance abuse and dependence disorders, eating disorders, somatoform disorders and medically unexplained conditions, and problems of memory and cognition. These complications are reflected in the DSM-5. PTSD contains diagnostic posttraumatic symptom clusters:

- Symptoms indicative of intrusive reliving of the trauma, the avoidance and numbing symptoms, and symptoms of increased autonomic arousal
- The episodic alternation between the avoidance and reliving symptoms is the result of dissociation
- Traumatic events are distanced and dissociated from usual conscious awareness in the numbing phase, only to return in the intrusive phase

Triggered by stimuli reminiscent of the trauma, these dissociated fragments of past experience return unbidden in the form of both psychological symptoms (amnesia, cognitive schemas of badness or worthlessness, intrusive images, dysregulated emotions) and somatoform symptoms (physical pain, physical numbing, intrusive sensations, and dysregulated autonomic arousal).

There are specific characteristics related to how a child experiences trauma, which are distinct from the way trauma is experienced by adults. Terr (1991) has classified a single incident trauma as a *Type I* trauma:

- Children may have full detailed memories because they are witnessing the event with more innocence and less preconceptions than adults
- At the same time, specific to their level of cognitive development, children may have inaccurate perceptions in their memories as they try to gain some mastery of the experience in retrospect and attempt to psychologically redo the event to make things right again

Some behaviors manifested in children with PTSD are: strongly visualized or otherwise repeatedly perceived memories; repetitive behaviors; trauma specific fears, and changed attitudes about people, aspects of life, and the future; regression to earlier behavior, such as thumb sucking, bed-wetting or clinging behavior; reluctance to go to bed because of nightmares and fears; fantasies that the disaster never happened; crying, screaming or withdrawal; refusal to attend and problems at school; and an inability to concentrate.

The creative arts therapy literature includes useful theoretical and practical information about working with trauma, and art made by patients who have experienced trauma. Avrahami (2006) describes visual art therapy as an integrative and unique approach, which is most appropriate for the multidimensional treatment of PTSD. The unique contribution of visual art therapy in the treatment of PTSD is expressed in three major areas:

(1) working on traumatic memories
(2) the process of symbolization–integration
(3) containment, transference, and countertransference

In this chapter, I will discuss developmental theory related to trauma and artwork made by patients who have experienced trauma, related to the areas of:

Abuse—sexual, physical, and emotional
Terrorism
Grief and Medical Illness
War
Natural disasters
Substance abuse related trauma

Abuse—Sexual, Physical, and Emotional

There are certain indicators in the artwork of victims of abuse. If clinicians are aware of these, they may be able to report the abuse, if necessary, and to offer supportive interventions. One of the saddest consequences of the pandemic lockdown is that victims of abuse are sheltering in place with their abusers. Children and adolescents living in abusive homes cherish school as a safe place and respite away from their abuser. Some victims of abuse make themselves physically ill by playing with medications or exposing themselves to something harmful in order to be brought to the hospital— another safe place and reprieve. Some victims may demonstrate psychiatric symptoms to be hospitalized for mental illness for this protection. Victims of domestic violence may do the same thing. Often, these patients become well known to the hospital staff, who become a good substitute family to them. If a victim is hospitalized on a behavioral health unit, especially repeatedly, social services will be involved, hopefully, getting them help and getting them out of the abusive situation. My experience has been that the staff on medical units may not respond as quickly to this person being a victim of abuse.

Sexual

Waller (1992) discusses art therapy with adult female incest survivors stating that there is valuable catharsis when using art medium and verbal expression of strong and long repressed emotion. Work in group allowed for cohesion as the women shared common experiences, and it allowed insight into the origins and present effects of serious problems.

In the artwork of victims of sexual abuse, this gingerbread person is common. This is a depersonalized human representation. It is spread out in a vulnerable position with no hands or feet to protect itself or run away. The stare is blank, the expression neutral. Exaggerated eyelashes are common

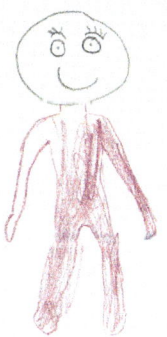

Figure 5.1 Gingerbread person typical in art of victims of sexual abuse

in the artwork of victims of sexual abuse. There is a clear cut off point between the head and the rest of the body. One can almost feel this image dissociating.

There are other identifiable characteristics of the art of victims of sexual abuse. Overly sexualized female images are common. Depersonalized or deprecating self-images are often seen or isolated self-images on a page. Tadpole humans are drawn by older children and adults, as if taking the body out of the picture literally or bodies without heads. There may be an appearance as if something is being inserted into the genital region. Placing an "X" over the genital area is common, as is crossing out the whole image represented. Projections and penis-like images are common.

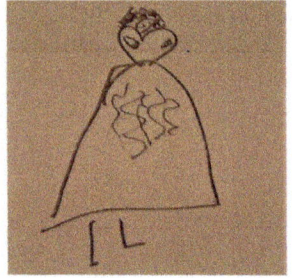

Overly sexualized female images

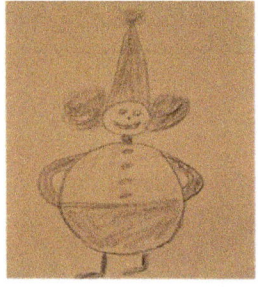

Depersonalized or deprecating self images

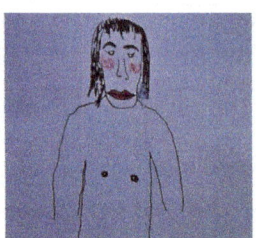

Depersonalized or deprecating self images

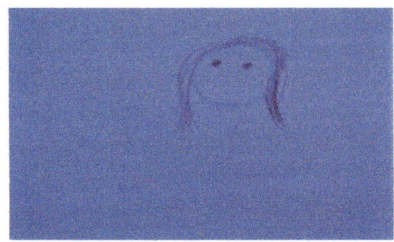

Isolated self images on a page

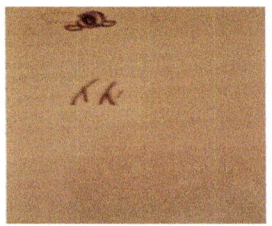

Isolated self images on a page

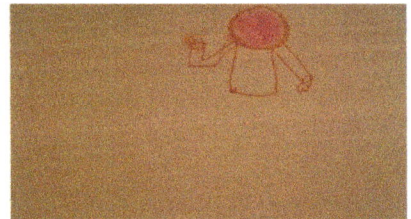

Isolated self images on a page;
crossed out face

Chart 5.1 Indicators of sexual abuse

Isolated self images on a page

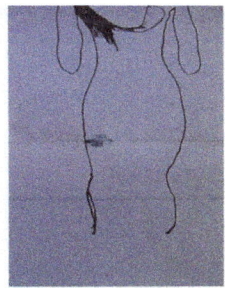

Bodies without heads

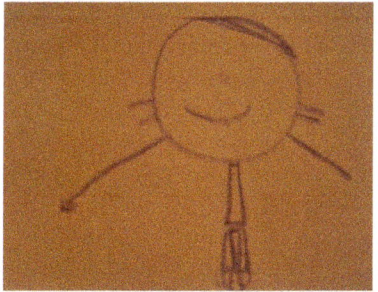

Appearance of insertions into
genital region

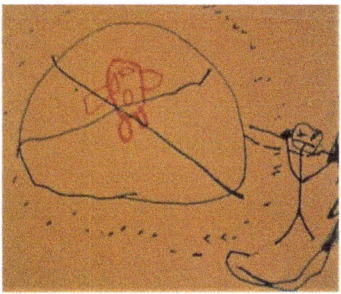

"X" over the genital area or crossing out
the whole image

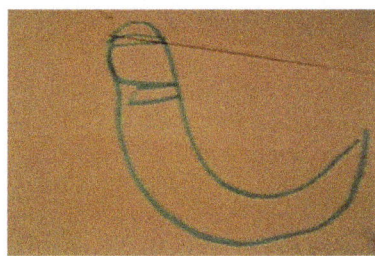

Projections and penis-like images

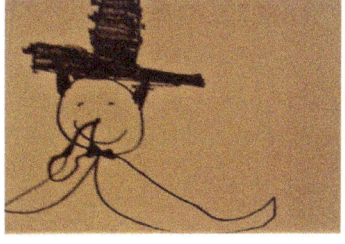

Projections and penis-like images

Chart 5.1 Continued

Sally

Sally found me on-line after many years had passed since I treated her and three of her siblings, Bobby, Marcy, and Alan, for sexual and physical abuse suffered in foster care during the 1980s. She was so happy to find me, and I was thrilled to hear from her and to hear that her life was going well, so we both thought. We reconnected through email.

> *Bobby and I were recently talking about you and how much fun we had during our group sessions.*

I would see two of the siblings, one before and one after, a sibling group session, and the other two the following week before and after the sibling group session. Sally told me that she was married to her partner of 15 years. They were raising two children—an adolescent girl, Angela, who was her brother's child born out of wedlock and a five-year-old boy, Leo, who was her partner's biological child, born within their marriage. Sally reported that she speaks with Bobby every day, although they had not seen each other in over 20 years. "He lives upstate and struggles, but he is a good person." Marcy was having a rough time at that point and had a long history of psychiatric hospitalizations. She was living in a shelter and had her two-year-old son taken away for neglect. "She really is a good Mom, just struggles." And then Alan. "Alan has spent more time in prison than out. I adopted his daughter who is now 14. I've had custody of her since she was two. So yes! I guess my family is pretty screwed up."

Sally said that she remembered the last time they saw me. I had gone to their home after their adoptive Mom died in a car wreck, but then their adoptive Dad broke off contact. "Did you hear what happened to us after that? It's been quite a ride!"

After the car accident in 1987, Sally explained to me that what no one knew until 1990 was that from the time they moved into the adoptive home, they were physically and sexually abused by the adoptive Dad, Sam, even when the adoptive Mom, Fran, was still alive. We both did not believe, or did not want to believe, that Fran knew of the abuse. After the car accident, the abuse got worse and was more frequent for all of them. Marcy finally broke and told her guidance counselor. Marcy, Sally, and Alan were placed into foster care. Bobby stayed with Sam because he was 17, but he was still being abused. Sally denied the abuse, as she usually did to maintain status quo, and was sent back home with Alan. They endured torture for another year.

> *At that point I went to my guidance counselor and told her that my sister was not lying. Sam spent seven years in prison. Alan has never been the same. He has been a drug addict since he was ten. He was beaten so badly by Sam. Marcy struggles. She was institutionalized from 11–21 and even after that. She was so badly hurt that I lied and said the abuse was not true. We are very close now, I feel horrible for the life she lived in hospitals. Such a crazy place!!*

Sally wanted to catch me up and let me know that the abuse had not just happened in foster care but in the adoptive home. She explained that it was hard for her as a little kid to talk about being abused in prior foster homes when it was still happening in her adoptive current home. And she was the sibling that had to testify in court in the suit her adoptive parents brought against the foster care family.

[Early in treatment, Sally drew this house. It does not sit on the black groundline with anal indulgent and urethral indulgent lines. The house has a scared face. Loop-like smoke swirls out of the chimney, urethral indulgent forms, towards the sun, most likely her abusive father. This is a good example at what looks like a typical latency period drawing but with several indicators of early abuse.]

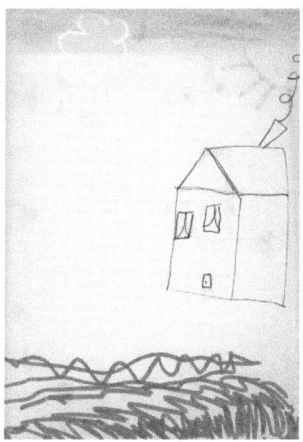

Figure 5.2 House drawn by Sally

I told her that when they missed their therapy session, I made many calls to the house with no response. I finally contacted Fran's Mom who told me what had happened. She seemed surprised that Sam did not tell me, but I got the feeling that she was being shut out, too. The only time Sam had called me after that time was when Marcy was about ten and ran into traffic in a suicide attempt. I told him she should be hospitalized for her own safety and begged him again to bring them back for therapy. At the time, he said that it was hard, but they were all getting by, day by day.

Sally often emailed me about Angela, her adopted daughter, who has a mood disorder and is often hospitalized or creating chaos in their home. "Teen age girls are tough." And for about two years, we had an ongoing email relationship. Then, Alan died of an overdose after getting out of jail. Sally was bereft that her little brother, whom she protected so many times over the years, had died. This tragedy brought back repressed memories that Sally had pushed down over time. She began to have terrible flashbacks and nightmares and became extremely anxious. Sally finally agreed to see me for art therapy, while continuing with her long-time therapist, and we agreed to collaborate.

Sally began to write down some of the flashbacks in a story called To Hell and Back. *They were terrible stories of abuse in every foster home, but the most horrific story she told was of how much Sam abused her. He would put a piece of wood against his bedroom door and rape her. He would tie her, naked, to a pole in the basement, leave her there, and then come back later, alone or with other men, and sexually abuse her. One of the most upsetting flashbacks to her (and to me) was this flashback from when she was fourteen:*

> *Sam decided he needed to make extra money (apparently he had accrued excessive gambling debts). He started cleaning offices in a professional building near the train station. He would leave the house at midnight and come home by 2:30–3 am on Tuesdays and Fridays. He did this a few times on his own. But*

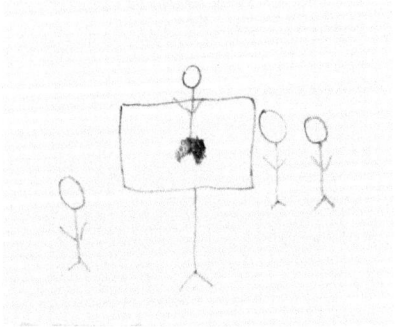

Figure 5.3a Being raped in Sam's room   *Figure 5.3b* Being used as a sex slave

very quickly told me I needed to help him clean. For the first few weeks it was OK; I was tired, but I never really slept much any way. I helped him clean this very brightly lit office; the office was all white and had slanted tables. I remember lots of eraser dust, and I can see the whole layout in my head.

One Friday late night we were on our way to clean. I was sleeping in the car. I woke up as the car stopped. We were at the train station. I was not sure what was going on. Within 10 minutes the car door opens, in comes two men. One is bald and husky and the other looks similar to Sam. I don't say anything. I feel them looking at me, I feel the hair on my arms standing. I just try and breathe. We get to the office, the men come in as well, I start to clean, but I am so distracted by them staring at me.

Sally went on to say that Sam told her to take her clothes off, and he tied her to a drawing table. The two men took off their clothes and sexually abused her. Sally realized that Sam was using her as a sex slave to pay off his gambling debts, and this then happened regularly. She remembered seeing blood all over the desk, which was so obvious in this brightly lit, white room. Sally was so demoralized by these experience that she did not even remember if she put her clothes on before getting into the car to go home.

In these pieces, Sally has drawn so lightly on the page that it is hard to even see what is going on. She is hardly visible on the bed. She is depersonalized to a stick figure. The light lines are like those that infants make. Sally is an infant whom no one took care of. She was robbed of that love and nurturing. She had a loving relationship with her partner, but, unfortunately, the recurring flashbacks and ongoing problems with Angela put a tremendous strain on their marriage. Sally no longer wanted to be intimate but would not share her flashbacks with her partner, even with my or her therapist's help. My hope was that if her partner knew what she had been through, they might be able to work things through. Now, she and her partner are separated, but living in the same house because of Leo.

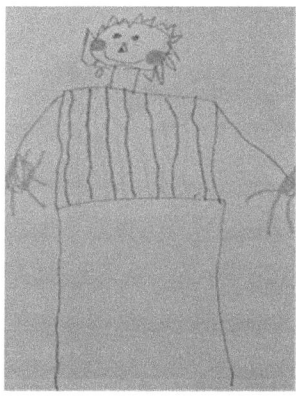

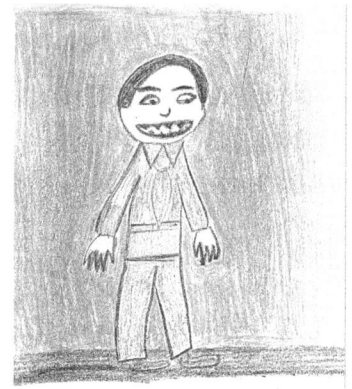

Figure 5.4a Typical spiky fingers during *Progressive Addition of Body Parts*

Figure 5.4b Adult who was physically abused

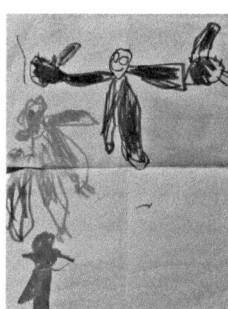

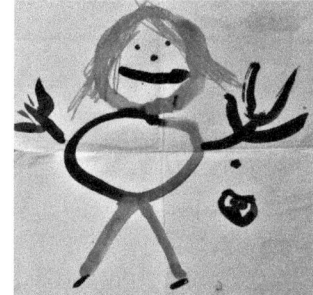

Figures 5.5a and b Latency period children who were physically abused

Physical

Dr. Kestenberg taught me a valuable lesson. She explained that if a child hits another child or an adult with a swatting motion using both hands, this is typical toddler behavior for expressing frustration or during a tantrum. If a child winds their arm back and then swings it forward forcefully with an open hand towards their victim, then this child is likely being hit, and possibly abused.

The artwork of victims of physical abuse will often have people with sharp teeth and spiky fingers. Caveat: When a child is going through DiLeo's stage of *Progressive Addition of Body Parts,* they will often draw spiky fingers because they are drawing the fingers with great attention to detail and concentration. However, if this is seen in the artwork of older children and adults, it could indicate physical abuse.

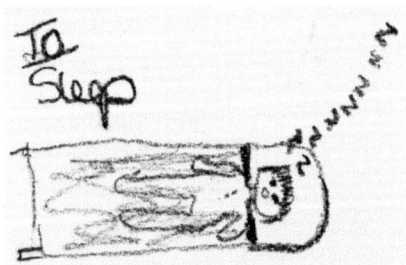

Figure 5.6 Sleeping with eyes open

Victims of abuse are vigilant, and this is often indicated in their artwork. This patient was sleep deprived due to being vigilant. Notice her ginger-bread person body and the line cutting her head off from her body and keeping her thinking cut off from her feelings and emotion.

Sometimes they will show the damage on the outside, and sometimes they will show the damage from the inside.

Patrick

Patrick was a 16-year-old boy, whom I treated in a special education school. Patrick had a conduct disorder and cognitive deficits. He lived with his father, who was physically abusive, which I suspected may account for his cognitive deficits. Patrick's Mom was deceased, and he had an older sister, who was married with kids and lived outside of the home. She was supportive of him but could not protect him. Patrick's drawings were typical of an adolescent in that he liked to play with perspective and tried to develop his own stylized art, Lowenfeld's Age of Decision and Rubin's Aestheticizing (see Figure 8). Figure 9. is interesting in that he is looking away (abuse victims often draw themselves as vigilant), and the back of his head is open and exposed. But there is an intricate network, anal indulgent, coming out of the top of his head—like radar. Urethral libidinal and urethral aggressive lines flow up the back of his head as if to say, "I wish I could run away, and this is who I am." And these lines protect some oral dotting within. Patrick's Mom had died when he was two years old, and he and his sister were left with an abuser. These lines point to a time in Patrick's life when attachment and separation/individuation were ripe. After doing this drawing, Patrick's father hit him in the head with a baseball bat causing concussion and breaking several teeth. After that, Patrick's sister took him to live with her.

Emotional

Emotional abuse is very insidious. Victims of emotional abuse wear their scars on the inside. They are anxious, hypervigilant, and eager to please. They

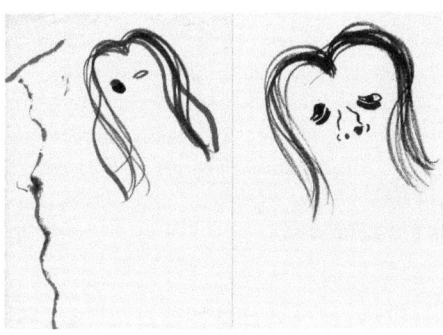

Figure 5.7a Black eyes and broken nose

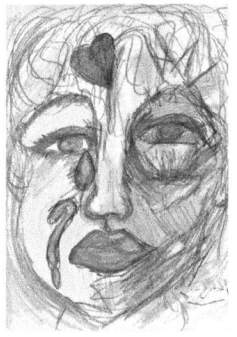

Figure 5.7b My inside scars

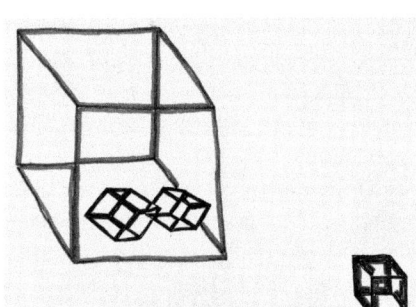

Figure 5.8 Perspective

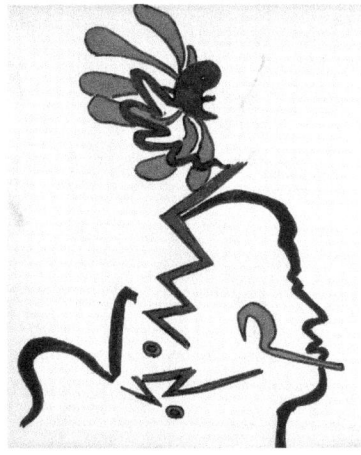

Figure 5.9 Stylized self-image

will sometimes make light of a situation so as not to draw the wrath of the abuser. This was the case with Avi.

Avi

Avi's Mom brought him to art therapy when he was nine years old. His Mom explained that she and her husband were seeking divorce but lived in the same house. Avi's father was emotionally abusive and would tell Avi that he was going to have a heart attack if Avi did not get him a cup of tea immediately, or that he was going to die, if Avi went to live with his mother. During the custody trial, I told this to the judge in his chambers, where he asked me to talk to him without parents or attorneys present. The judge took a few deep breaths and looked me straight in the eye saying,

"I'd rather someone smacked me across the face than say something like that to me." I commented that he made that statement, not me.

Avi's attempts at lightening the mood were apparent in the way he would be seeming to be entertaining me in sessions, even when I was pushing heavy issues, like divorce, with him. I owe a great debt to Marge Heegard and her Drawing Out Your Feelings Series of workbooks. I have used them often and with many children and highly recommend them to anyone working with children. They are well organized and structured to be used in sessions with children and adolescents and support resolution of hard times. One of the activities I had Avi complete was "Why do people get married? Why do people get divorced?"

Avi's images are typical of latency period children. Avi's verbal responses to both are very reasonable, but to the first about why people get married, his images tell more. The wedding celebrant looks like a Bishop or Cardinal—a nod to the sanctity of marriage, perhaps. But this clergyman is smoking a big cigar diminishing that sacred ceremony. The bride and groom have no faces, which makes this funny image, not so funny as you realize the lack of connection he feels to his parents. There's a certain transparency in the image, which is more common in the art of younger children, but it might be Avi's letting me see through some of the façade of his parents into who they are and how they have left their scars.

In the second image about why people get divorced, the people are folded out, identified as typical by Lowenfeld for this age. But they have no faces, like the bride and groom. Also typical for this age, Avi is showing action of the judge's gavel with an arrow. The judge's stand is filled in with anal libidinal lines. Avi did have digestive problems when he was anxious, and in addition to all the anxiety he was feeling at home, Avi was nervous about possibly having to testify.

Ultimately, Avi's Mom got residential custody and moved them out of their house to a new one, and the judge recommended that his Dad get into therapy or take a parenting class. When they were not living together, Avi and his Dad had a warmer relationship in which Avi felt more relaxed interacting with his Dad.

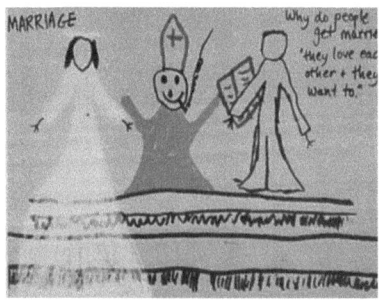
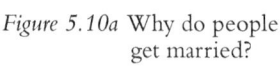
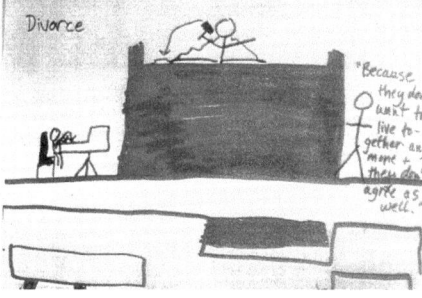

Figure 5.10a Why do people get married?

Figure 5.10b Why do people get divorced?

Terrorism

Terrorism is an all-too-common phenomenon in our current world. It comes in many forms and usually takes victims. Whether it is religious extremists or White supremacists, it happens on every continent and breeds hate and division.

Jones (1997) wrote about the use of art therapy after an incident of domestic terrorism. On April 19, 1995, the most devastating act of domestic terrorism ever perpetrated in the USA occurred in Oklahoma City, Oklahoma. In the immediate aftermath, there was a dearth of mental health professionals experienced in dealing with the sequela of violent, deadly trauma. The extensiveness of the tragedy, which included the destruction of the Federal Building and the death of 169 people and injury to another 500, was unparalleled. Due to considerable clinical experience in dealing with violent trauma, treating PTSD patients, organizing critical incident response teams, and availability, Jones was asked to spearhead the local Indian Health Science mental health team. He describes the experience of providing clinical services to more than 120 victims and their families in the six months following the bombing.

The art therapy technique that Jones employed with survivors and families was using charcoal on large sheets of paper. Participants were instructed to cover the paper with charcoal and then use a kneaded eraser to pull out images to express their feelings of pain, anger, sadness, loss, and helplessness. The experience helped participants pull out buried feelings—a metaphor to help them grieve their family or friends buried by the explosion. I have used Jones' technique with patients, and it is very effective for pulling out feelings of trauma for the purpose of looking at and possibly resolving associated issues.

After the terrorist attack on the World Trade Center (WTC) on 9/11/01, creative arts therapists were recognized as valued and needed counselors alongside other mental health professionals. Creative arts therapists in the New York area were called upon to provide trauma debriefing, answer crisis phones, counsel bereaved family members, advise school personnel about how children might react to the trauma and how it might be seen in their art, work with airline personnel, and work with firefighters and the bereaved families of lost rescue workers.

Thousands of traumatized New Yorkers experienced the terrorist attacks of 9/11/01 firsthand, making recovery more difficult. The families of SoHo and neighboring communities live near the WTC. Many families were forced out of their homes either due to recovery efforts or because of damage caused by the attack. Residents of that neighborhood experienced the loss of family members and friends.

The Children's Museum of the Arts, located in SoHo, is a community center where children and families create together through involvement with the visual and performing arts. In an effort to offer a neighborhood center for families to collectively process the events of 9/11/01 and to heal as a

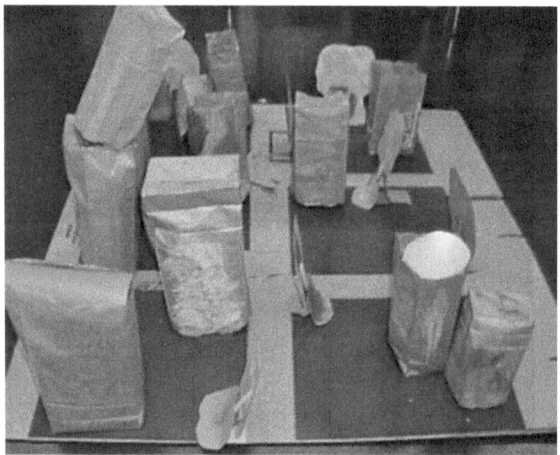

Figure 5.11 Young children's response to 9/11/01

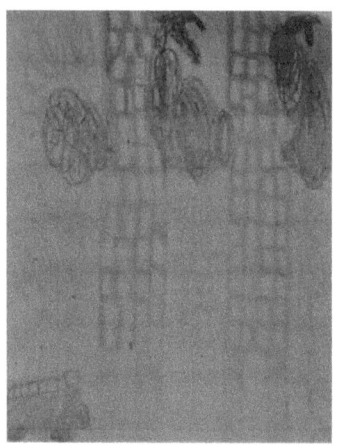

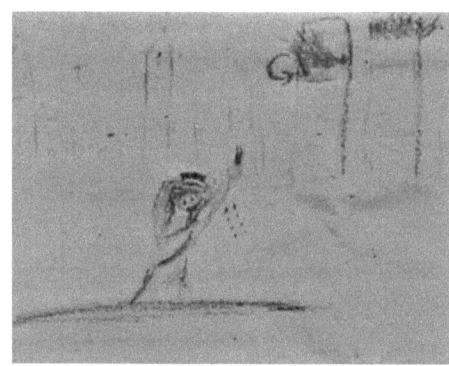

Figure 5.12 WTC on 9/11/01   *Figure 5.13* The Statue of Liberty cries

community, the museum's director and staff reached out to its members and others in the community through the use of art and art projects. I organized *Operation Healing* so that art services could be provided for all age groups, including parents (Gonzalez-Dolginko, 2002). The younger children made a three-dimensional map of the area. As Terr (1991) points out, children will sometimes want to believe that the traumatic incident never happened, or they will make up a different ending. Typical to their age, the younger children made towers and many of them had antennae on top, like the WTC. They also included helicopters in the layout because they wanted to believe that helicopters rescued people, even though it did not happen.

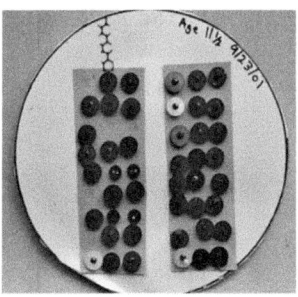

Figure 5.14a 11½ year old's WTC

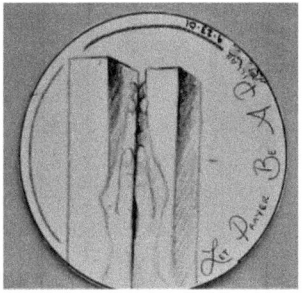

Figure 5.14b Older adolescent's WTC

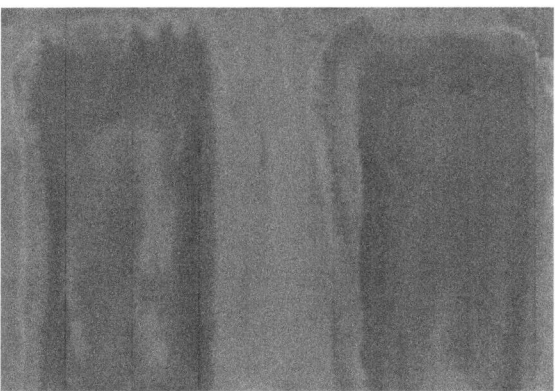

Figure 5.15 Adult's memory of 9/11/01

Per Terr (1991), Latency Period children drew very specific images of the witnessed scene, and this image even shows how smoky it was at ground level. Children typically demonstrate emotion in their art at this age, such as the Statue of Liberty's distressed look and crying.

Older children and adolescents made mandalas, many of which had hopeful messages. It is typical of this age that placing hope and love in religious beliefs can support healing. Young adolescents were more concrete and organized with the representations in their mandalas, Lowenfeld's *Age of Reason*. Older adolescents' representations demonstrated Piaget's *Formal Operational* stage and Lowenfeld's *Age of Decision*.

The adults used the opportunity of the parent group, which I facilitated, to process many of the emotions that they felt they could not express in front of their children or friends who lost family members. The group offered them relief and a safe place. Their images were light on the page giving a feeling of helplessness. These images were also ghost-like perhaps representing people, objects, and buildings that are no longer there. In Figure 5.15 dense anal lines fill the ghost-like towers as if trying to hang on to them when all control is gone. Many of them drew one tower standing, a common memory reported by most adult witnesses with whom I worked.

Grief/Medical Illness

Grief

Grief and medical illness have presented together in my clinical experience. A patient who had an organ transplant disagreed with me when I pointed out that he was going through the stages of dying (Kübler-Ross, 1969) because he had not died. I pointed out to him that he was grieving his old life and organ. We reviewed his art together, and I pointed out spiritual images, images of transformation, and side-by-side images of dying and rebirth. Then he could understand that his grief did not have to be related only to death.

When diagnosed with a terminal illness, one is faced with mortality and begins to grieve. Kübler-Ross (1969) outlines five stages of loss and grief as denial, anger, bargaining, depression, and acceptance. In a later work, Kübler-Ross and Kessler (2005) clarify that these classically adopted stages are not necessarily sequential or all universally experienced. These stages are a commonality to people grieving.

There is significant literature documenting the use of creative arts therapies towards healing with cancer patients (Nainis, 2005; Nainis et al., 2006; Zammit, 2001), and some with chronic illness (Wadeson, 2003; Nishida & Strobino, 2005).

Feen-Calligan, McIntyre, and Sands-Goldstein, M. (2009) review the history of dollmaking that is relevant to art therapy, and the application of dolls as therapeutic media in clinical and educational settings. The authors describe their experiences using dollmaking in the resolution of grief, in professional identity construction, and in community service, and they discuss benefits of dollmaking in clinical practice, as well as for personal awareness.

Hailey

Hailey, who is 11, lost her grandmother to whom she was very close. Her Mom sought art therapy for her because she felt Hailey was not grieving Mimi. Mom had taken Hailey to the bereavement groups offered by hospice, had the school counselors speak with her, and took her to therapists who use words in their treatment. None of it was working for Hailey. She would not talk about Mimi in any of these settings. She was becoming increasingly depressed and expressing feelings that she wanted to die so that she could be with Mimi. This is a difficult age to lose a dear one, and there is no true cognition that death is a permanent state.

I suggested to her Mom that Hailey bring some pictures of Mimi. Interestingly, Hailey brought photos with Mimi only, and they were pictures from when Mimi was dying. Hailey did not have much to say but was thrilled to work with all the fun art supplies in my office. I suggested that we make a frame for the photos, and she agreed, creating a frame that was typically preadolescent with stickers, sparkles, and lots of detail. Still, Hailey did not spontaneously offer any information about Mimi but did answer my questions. When I asked Hailey if she talked to Mimi with her heart, she looked at me as if I were mad and shook her head "No" vehemently.

Her Mom had told me that she is an anxious kid and that her anxiety had increased after Mimi's death. She also has trouble sleeping. I asked Hailey about her anxiety and what she understands about it from other therapies that she has had. She was not forthcoming with any information. I asked her if she knows what a worry doll is. "They don't work!!" I acknowledged her comment but suggested that we make a Mimi doll using the worry doll kit that I have. Hailey was intrigued by the idea and made a list of supplies she wanted to get at the crafts store for Mimi's clothing. The next week, we started in, and Hailey spontaneously told me stories about Mimi. When we had some mishaps with gluing on the tiny eyes, I verbalized an apology to Mimi for the problem. Hailey giggled and thought that was funny. By the third week that we were working on the Mimi doll, I had heard many Mimi stories, and Hailey transformed mishaps into announcing that Mimi was going to have some surgery to correct the problems. During the "surgery," Hailey kept checking in with Mimi asking her if she were doing OK. By the time we were finished, Mimi was a very glamorous doll, and Hailey was a proud dollmaker. She took Mimi home and put her in a special place in her room, and I suspect that she talks to her with her heart.

Medical Illness

Medical illnesses are classified as acute, chronic, and/or terminal diseases. Physical health issues affect almost everyone at some point in their lives. People may develop an illness themselves or indirectly experience illness through a friend or family member's condition.

Buday (2013) speaks to benefits that art therapy may offer to support the emotional, psychosocial, and spiritual well-being of hospice patients by using imagery and symbolism to communicate challenging emotions; gaining self-empowerment through the engagement of making art and reflecting on the resulting product; and offering a non-threatening means to explore thoughts and feelings.

Terrence

Terrence, a 37-year-old gay man, was diagnosed with AIDS. Through art therapy and engaging with his visual images, Terrence was able to reflect upon issues of shame, sadness, alienation, lack of connection with his family, grief, and facing death. Terrence dealt with some issues of anger and abandonment and then focused more on the present. Terrence was excited about being accepted into a clinical trial. In his image, seen below, he writes the word, EXCITEMENT, in red, which stands out and may be reflective of the blood virus. Because we had been focused on issues from his early childhood, this piece has oral, anal, urethral, and inner genital lines in its composition.

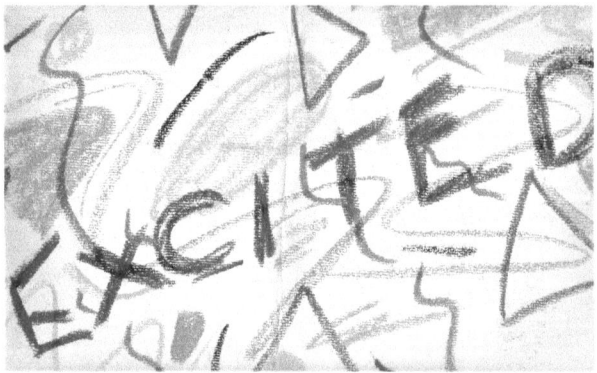

Figure 5.16 Terrence is excited about participating in a clinical trial

Terrence includes several urethral aggressive signature lines throughout the piece that he identified in another piece as a Kaposi's sarcoma. Oral dotting prevails throughout the image. It seems to be reflecting the great sense of loss and separation that he was feeling. He was hopeful because of some medical treatments that were slowing down his loss of t-cells, but his count was so low at that point, that he would not see a reversal of his disease. Throughout his art therapy treatment, Terrence was able to go deeply into the process of dying. His imagery allowed him to review and resolve issues so that he could face his terminal illness.

War

Wars cover the world, and many of them are ongoing for years and lead to death, destruction, heinous acts of violence, suffering, and refugeeism. Although I have not worked with veterans, many creative arts therapists have, and I acknowledge the trauma they have endured.

Lobban (2014) argues for the efficacy of art therapy for veterans. Art therapy groups with a thematic analysis approach supported veterans' understanding of the benefit of art therapy. Lobban also explores the neuro-biological processes involved in PTSD and examines how art therapy might assist recovery on a structural level.

Baker (2006) describes a refugee program in Chicago. Mental health clinics can use creative art therapies as a means of reaching out to war refugees in their communities who may not respond to traditional talk therapy. In this case, the use of quilting and other artwork was utilized by the staff at Chicago Health Outreach to assist displaced Bosnians to cope with their war-related trauma and integration into their new environment in the USA. It can be difficult to reach refugee populations within a community whose culture and language are different from the majority, but finding other means of communicating can make a real difference for these individuals as they find safety and understanding by working on and sharing special creative projects.

In the mid-1990s, I was asked to be on the advisory board of the Children's Museum of the Arts (CMA) in SoHo, New York, because I was a specialist in children's art. The founder and then, director, Kathleen Schneider, was passionate about the museum and children making art. I remained on this advisory board for ten years. This was a wonderful and memorable professional experience. My advice was originally sought because they wanted my help curating a few shows of the artwork of children from the former Yugoslavia when they were in the throes of war. CMA had acquired the children and adolescent art from Physicians without Borders, other human rights groups, and a professional soccer player who was originally from the former Yugoslavia. Each group wisely brought art supplies with them to offer healing activities when working with children and adolescents in refugee camps. CMA's director wanted copy, written by a child development specialist, that would accompany the artwork and that would explain about war and the refugees fleeing the country to NYC school children coming to the show.

What immediately occurred to me as I approached this task was that many NYC children have been exposed to excessive violence and may not be as shocked as CMA's director thought they would be. A particular piece came to mind.

This piece came to my attention through one of my art therapy students who was working on a community-building initiative through the New York Police Department (NYPD). The directive was to draw something bad that happened in your community and what you did about it. This young child drew their grandfather being shot. Notice that this child in the early part

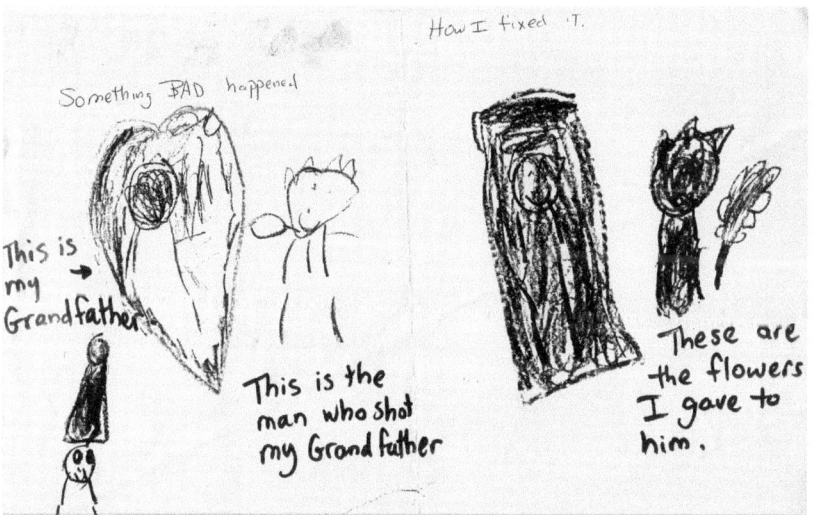

Figure 5.17 Something bad that happened in my neighborhood and what I did about it

of Lowenfeld's *Schematic Stage,* encloses his grandfather in a heart to protect him from the gunshot. The gunman has a smile on his face and looks like a tadpole, which would be more typical of Lowenfeld's *Pre-schematic Stage.* The child may experience some regression due to having seen such a traumatic event. This can also be seen with the significant amount of anal denseness coloring on the right side of the page. The child's grandfather lived, and he is bringing him flowers in the hospital. But this is certainly something horrible witnessed by a NYC child.

Nevertheless, I worked with the staff of CMA to develop an informative experience that was sensitive to social and emotional issues. Viewing this art was an honor.

My observations of this war art were that it was well executed, regardless of age, leading me to believe that these children had formal art education, most likely in their schools. There were many images of people fleeing because they had to leave their homes and of a mother's love and precious things in the home left behind. And there were images of death and destruction. The images from the refugee camps were all interiors, as if they were protecting themselves in what were their new, but temporary, homes.

My reputation as a researcher of children's war art spread, and at an *American Art Therapy Association* conference, I was approached by a young man from Kuwait. Yaqub al Dashtir was an art teacher for children in Kuwait from kindergarten through high school. He had collected children's art in Kuwait during the occupation and then after the liberation and was writing about this process and the children's art for his doctoral dissertation. Yaqub asked me if I would be a reader of his dissertation and offer some analysis of the art. Again, I felt honored.

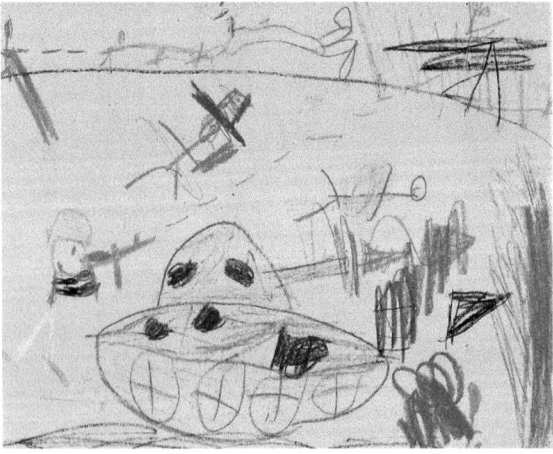

Figure 5.18 A young child's view of the war in the former Yugoslavia

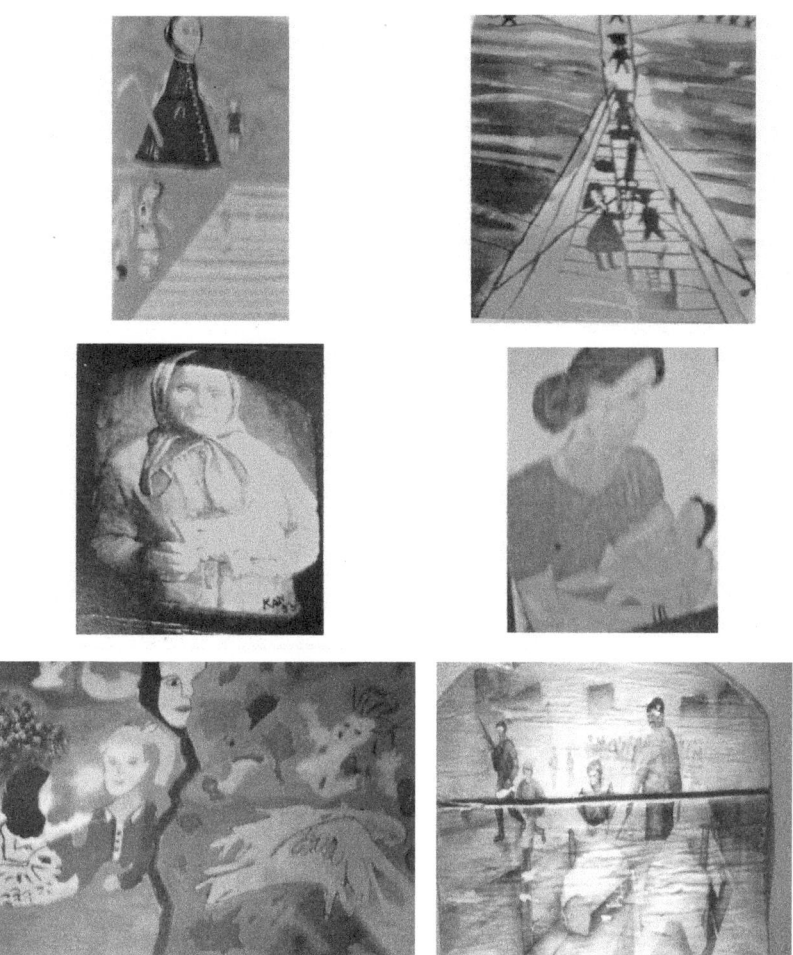

Chart 5.2 Child and adolescent art from the war in the former Yugoslavia

The art was beautiful, and Yaqub informed me that children in Kuwait do have formal art training throughout school. Having reviewed and studied the artwork of the Bosnian refugees offered me an interesting standard of comparison. The Kuwaiti children remained in their occupied city, as opposed to the Bosnian refugees who had to flee. There are far more images of atrocities in the Kuwaiti children's art because they saw violence in the street, like public executions. Because they were sequestered to their homes and many of their brothers and fathers were jailed, there were many images of internal spaces. Trying to prevail against being occupied, one of the prevalent characteristics in the art include a sense of nationalism—the Kuwaiti flag, outlines of the country itself with someone kissing it.

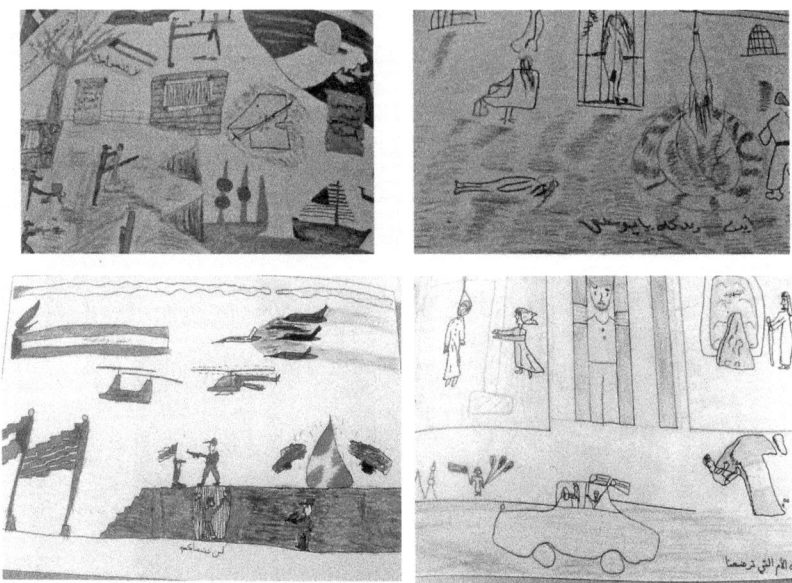

Chart 5.3 Child and adolescent art from the War in Kuwait

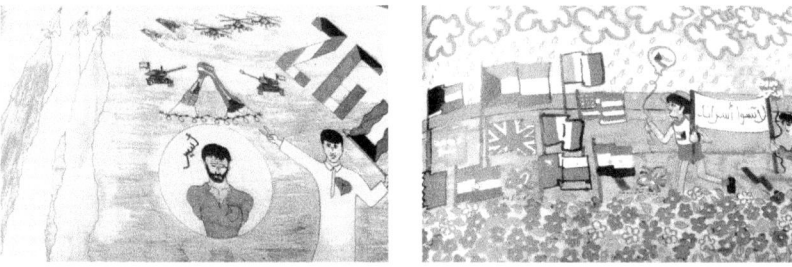

Figure 5.19a A boy draws *Kuwait is free*   *Figure 5.19b* A girl draws *Kuwait is free*

The pictures drawn after the liberation from occupation were joyful, most featuring the flags of Kuwait and the nations of the UN forces that liberated them.

Viewing the art developmentally, images that are typical of children in the latency period emerge. My assumption was that the jets and tanks were drawn by boys, and the flowers and rainbow streamers, of Kuwait's national colors, were drawn by girls, and Yaqub confirmed my assumptions.

Natural Disasters

Natural disasters are devastating to people and communities. What can one do if the earth is shaking or heavy rain is bombarding your home for three days straight leaving feet of rain? Power and connectivity are disrupted, sometimes for weeks or months. There is a feeling of helplessness and isolation, disorientation, and despair. People die. Homes and cities are destroyed. There is some useful literature on creative arts therapies with people following natural disasters.

Chang (2005) wrote of the use of drama therapy after a 7.3 magnitude earthquake which occurred on September 21, 1999, in Taiwan. It destroyed more than 100,000 houses, causing 2,294 deaths and 8,737 injuries. In the aftermath of the earthquake, a great number of social workers and cultural workers travelled to Nantou County and Taichung County of central Taiwan, the epicenter of the earthquake, to assist the survivors. Therapeutic workshops of the *Truth Good Beauty Human Potential Centre* were held in more than eight elementary schools and junior high schools to help those children who suffered the loss of family members and to assist those who suffered from PTSD.

In some villages of central Taiwan, local people are quite conservative, and they find Western concepts of psychotherapy or therapeutic theatre quite foreign. Suffering from PTSD, many people would rather seek help from a shaman or through an indigenous ritual than consult a psychotherapist or social workers. Under such circumstances, it becomes a challenging task for therapists and social workers to break the ice and win the trust of village people.

Andruk (1996) is an art therapist who needed to process her own trauma from an earthquake so that she could better help patients with psychosis process their trauma. To deal with her needs during the three weeks after the earthquake they had all experienced, the author created her own art in a series of small collages. They were useful in dealing with the nervousness and edginess she felt going to work at the epicenter each day, the impact of seeing the damage created, and the seemingly endless road winding through two dust-fed valleys between home and work.

Roje (1995) worked with 25 children at the site of an elementary school in the area hardest hit by the Los Angeles earthquake in 1994 and offers clinical observations about issues most relevant to the trauma, symptomatology, and defenses exhibited by children during treatment after doing art therapy interventions with latency aged children telling their earthquake story in words and in pictures. By processing the art, the children were able to explore their current and repetitive thoughts, and to work through their feelings toward the resolution of the trauma and help them return to normal functioning.

Although I am aware of several art therapists who worked using art with survivors of both Hurricane Katrina and Superstorm Sandy, I am unable to find anything that they may have published regarding this. I do know from students and supervisees doing this work after Superstorm Sandy that many of the neighborhoods affected by the storm were also neighborhoods that had been impacted after the terror attacks of 9/11/01, and their PTSD symptoms were exacerbated. I am sure that a comparison of artwork gathered from each would be an interesting study.

Tara

Tara was ten years old when she and her Mom were in a car together, and the road collapsed under them during an earthquake. Tara had been a gifted student, artist, and violinist. After this tragedy, she developed a seizure disorder and became nonverbal. It was truly one of the most fascinating examples of a conversion reaction that I have seen in my practice. Her Mom brought her to me for art therapy because she was not speaking. Tara was also under the care of neurologists who wanted her Mom to medicate her. Tara's EEGs indicated that her brain was in a constant state of seizures, but her Mom was reluctant to medicate her. I suggested that she do so because the constant seizures were causing Tara to seem as if she were a baby—drooling, eyes staring, and no speech. I also explained that the constant seizures could be causing neurological damage. The medication helped the seizures to subside, and Tara's personality began to reconstitute.

I cannot take credit for a cure through remarkable art therapy, but I did witness and assist Tara as she went through developmental stages towards her healing. Tara's original artwork was like infant art with scribbles eventually becoming lines and forms, per the KAP. She did the art frenetically and often would rip the paper in the process or tear it after she was done. She would make several pieces in one session, often crumbling to the floor afterwards as if exhausted.

Slowly, Tara became more deliberate with her art, like a pre-schematic child and forms emerged, as language returned. I often play the scribble game with children of this age to connect with them (Winnicott, 1971b). Very often, even though it seems like a simple game, what children see in the scribbles gives the art therapist insight into their issues. The scribbles that Tara presented to me were similar to the chaotic art she did when first entering treatment. I would try to organize the scribble as best as I could. I made Tara's scribble into a little girl elephant trainer. I did not do this consciously, but I think I was giving Tara the message that she can train this "elephant" of seismic energy that she was feeling in her head. After this, her scribbles were less complex.

Eventually, she was weaned off the medication, and she was the old Tara. She and her Mom moved to an area that was not in an earthquake zone, and she successfully returned to school and music lessons. Tara sent me a picture that is a perfect preadolescent rendering. The images are realistic and precise with an awareness of

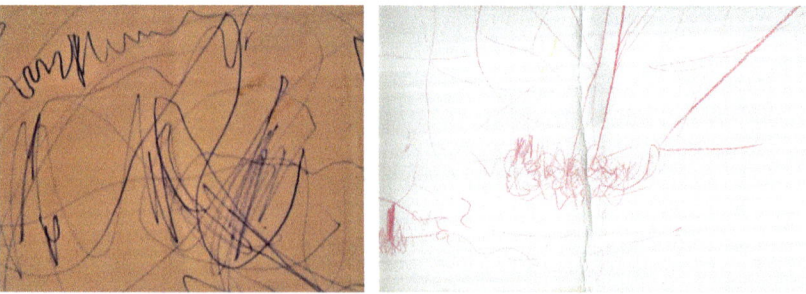

Figure 5.20 Tara's art made while constantly seizing

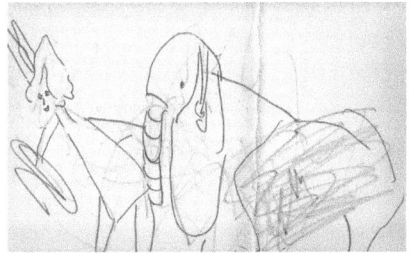

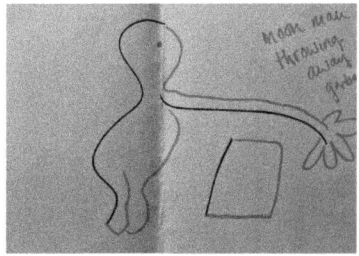

Figure 5.21a Beth makes Tara's scribble into a little girl elephant trainer

Figure 5.21b Simpler scribble

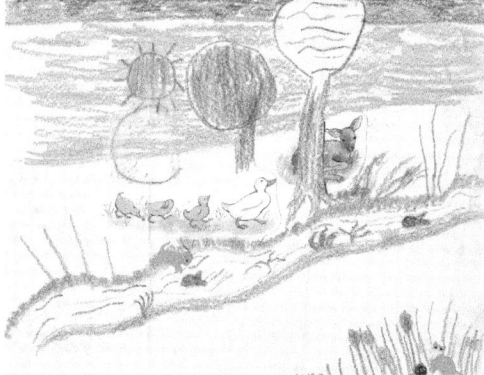

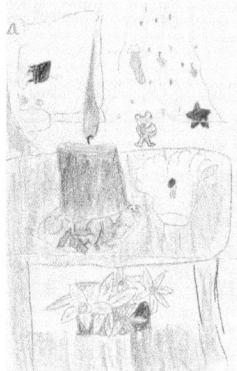

Figures 5.22 Tara's art after her recovery

perspective and proportion. The addition of the stickers is typical of girls this age. Yet, Tara demonstrated some of her artistic skill by cutting the sticker of the deer in half to carefully place it around the tree giving the impression that the deer is lying down behind the tree. Tara also sent me a beautiful Christmas card, which is a nicely rendered piece for her age.

Substance Abuse Related Trauma

Addiction is at an alarmingly high rate in the USA. Societal and economic stress lay fertile soil for substance abuse, thus compounding trauma. Skeffington and Browne (2014) remark that the literature regarding the efficacy of treatment programs for post-trauma pathologies is prolific. Yet, little attention is paid to the treatment of resistant and complex trauma. While therapists recognize that a trauma history needs to be considered and explored with most patients, the authors feel that therapists must hone their skills at identifying complex trauma. Avoidance of distressing thoughts, feelings and images can manifest in a range of symptoms and behaviors other than PTSD, with substance abuse high on that list. The creative arts therapies employ the language of imagery, which can allow expression where conversational language has failed. Before therapists can treat any issues that patients bring to therapy, they must address addictions.

Donna

Donna was in her mid-30s when she entered art therapy. She was addicted to heroin and wanted to go to rehab. Donna cried as she told me that she does not even feel high anymore when she uses but is physically dependent. Her routine was that she went to work at her Civil Service job every day, scored heroin on her way home from work, shared it with her boyfriend, Joe, and then cooked dinner for them both even though he had been sitting home all day watching TV. In this picture, Donna's back is to us as Joe shoots up with a smile on his face. The only color in the piece is red at the injection sight and blue on the table where she cooks dinner—both things that she does to take care of him.

Donna had reported her addiction to Human Resources (HR) so that she could get into a top-ranked rehabilitation program with which her HR had an affiliation. She was going to marry Joe so that he could have access to this program rather than going to a program in a municipal hospital. I tried to discourage her from doing this and to just worry about herself as her therapy continued. When Donna mentioned something to her HR counselor that she had discovered in our treatment, he asked her why I was treating her when, ethically, I should not be treating her while she was still addicted. At her next session, Donna asked me this. I explained to her that I was treating her addiction to Joe so that she could then work on her addiction to heroin. This made sense to Donna, and she made the decision to not marry him and enter the rehab that HR offered her alone with a successful outcome.

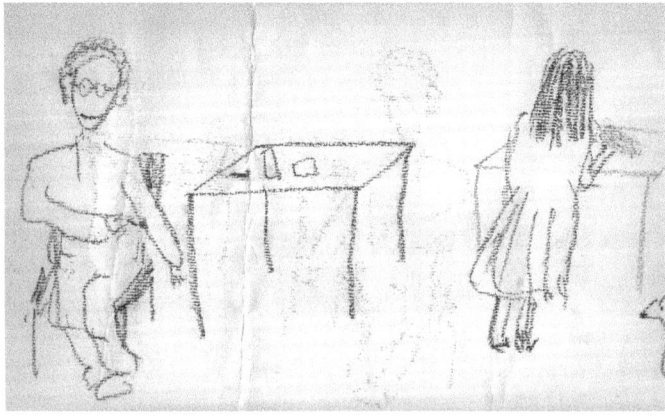

Figure 5.23 Donna cooks dinner while Joe shoots up

Many treatments for addictions have a low success rate, and complex trauma exacerbates this. Many seasoned clinicians in addictions will insist that *12-Steps* programs offer the best outcomes. Moos and Timko (2008) discuss the efficacy of *12-Steps* and other self-help groups, often called mutual help or support groups. They feel these groups are an important component of the system of care for patients with substance abuse disorders. Individuals make more visits to self-help groups for help with their own or family member's substance use and psychiatric problems than to all mental health professionals combined. The authors indicate that as many as 9% of adults in the USA have been to an Alcoholics Anonymous (AA) meeting at some time in their lives, and more than 3% have been to a meeting in the prior year (Room and Greenfield 1993). Moreover, many substance abuse treatment service providers have adopted *12-Steps* techniques in treatment, and most of them refer patients to self-help groups. Patients with addictions have high rates of posttreatment relapse and often require additional episodes of specialized care. The authors found that self-help groups improve the likelihood of achieving and maintaining remission and may reduce the need for further professional care.

Horay (2006) acknowledges the value and importance of *12-Steps* programs. The author suggests differing approaches that have been developed within the area of addictions which could support the gains of those programs. Motivational interviewing, coupled with therapeutic artmaking and enacted in a stages-of-change model, adds dimension to exploring the ambivalence experienced throughout the initial stages of substance abuse treatment. This approach promotes self-efficacy rather than confronting denial or highlighting one's powerlessness over alcohol and drugs and seems to have some success against relapse.

Feen-Calligan (2007) brings attention to an all-too-common and increasing phenomenon in addictions treatment. Many patients are brought into the hospital and need to be detoxed before they can be placed on a behavioral health unit. This is really the first stop in addictions treatment. The author documents the lack of literature concerning detoxification from chemical addiction and suggests that art therapists need to re-evaluate their services for this population, beginning in the detoxification phase of treatment.

Giving this some thought, I seized an opportunity with a young patient, who had just been admitted to our behavioral health unit after he was detoxed from opiates. He announced to the group that his father had taken pictures of him on the detox unit with tubes and IVs coming out from all over his body. I asked him if he had the pictures. He said that he did not. I strongly suggested that he get those pictures from his Dad and put them up in his hospital room and his bedroom when he finally went home and then continue to look at them every time he wanted to use again. The young man heard me and understood where I was coming from, and we both acknowledged how powerful those images were, hopefully preventing relapse.

Addictions counselors say that a person's development stops at the age they are when they start using. Most of the art that I have seen done by patients with addictions resembles that of adolescents. The imagery of patients with addictions demonstrates oral dependency. Some of the common symbols or

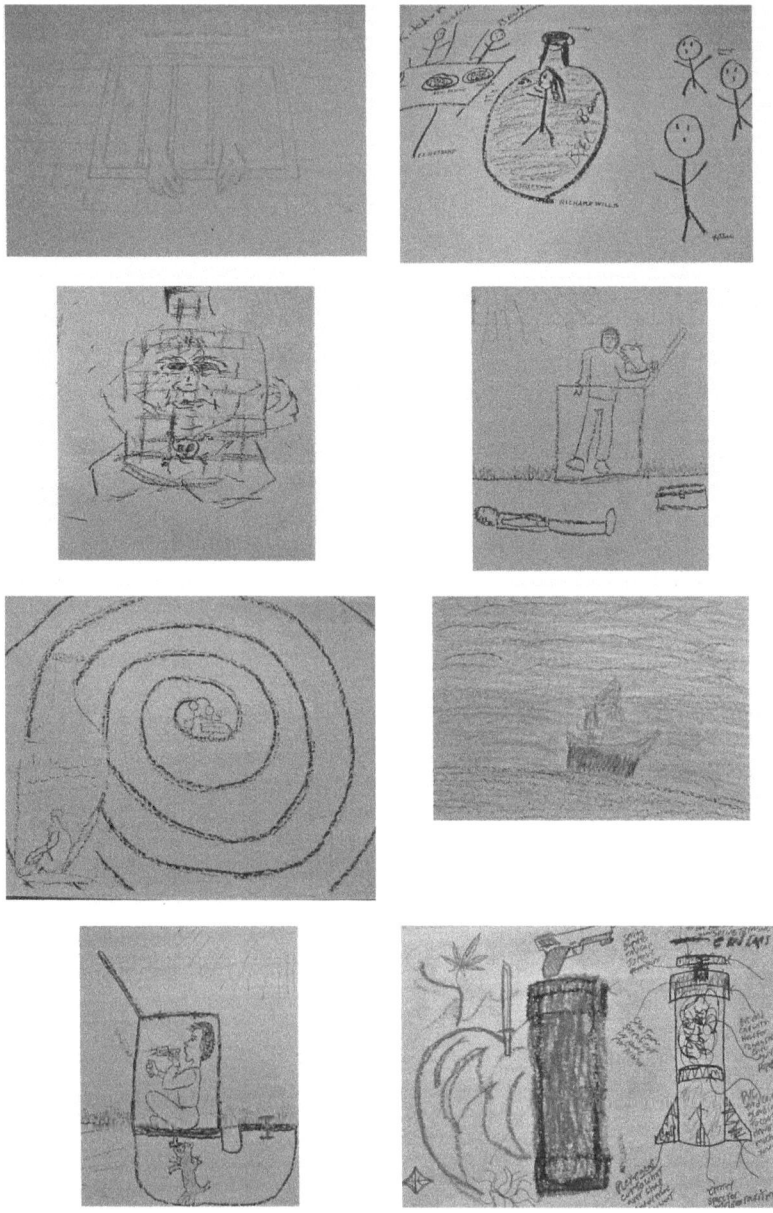

Chart 5.4 Imagery related to addictions

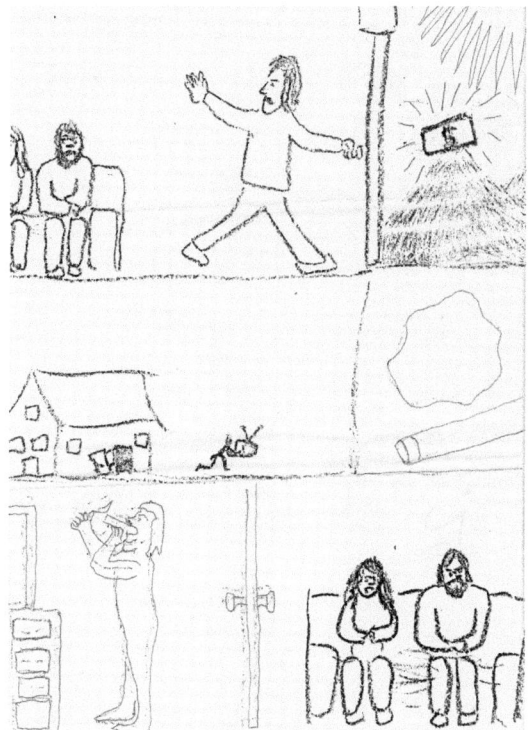

Figure 5.24 Fighting with my parents about my using crack

characteristics of art by patients with addictions are that they are trapped or imprisoned, often in a bottle. Spirals and water imagery are common. And, as would be expected, imagery related to the use of drugs and alcohol.

Imagery related to the disruption in their family lives is also common.

Kathy

Kathy was in her 50s when I began working with her on a behavioral health unit. She was a warm and kind person but could not stop drinking. She had lost custody of her children, her driver's license, and her nursing license due to her alcoholism. Kathy had periods of sobriety, sometimes lasting a few years, and even regained her nursing license, but she always relapsed. Trying to make sense of this, Kathy did an art piece trying to figure this out. It has a very latency period/school-aged feel to it. She represents recognizable people (although stick figures) and objects and tells a story. Kathy divides up the page to tell her stories of shame, love, and peace. Shame represents mistakes she made as a nurse because she was drunk. Love is the most peaceful part of her story, but it is sparse. In this part of Kathy's story, she is holding one of her babies with preadolescent hearts floating around. But the sun image overwhelms the composition

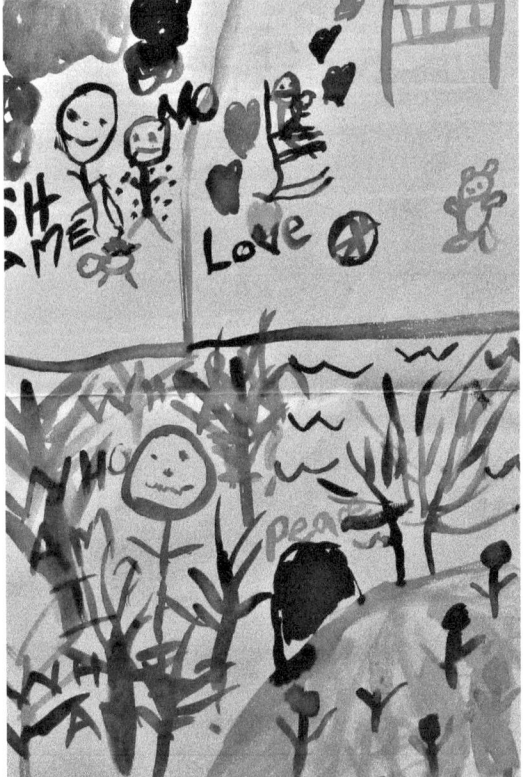

Figure 5.25 Kathy trying to make sense of her life of drinking

and may represent her father who was a rageful alcoholic and influenced her life signifi-
cantly. The crib looks more like a barred window—Kathy had spent time in jail for a
DWI. The teddy bear is the most developed form in her picture but looks very lonely.
And her peace story is anything but peaceful. Her facial expression is pained. There is
a black mass in the middle that may be a grave. The six flowers may represent Kathy,
her husband, and their four children. And they are on a slope that is going downhill,
like her life. She writes the question "Who am I?" as birds that look like urethral
aggressive signature lines float overhead. Kathy's early development and childhood was
very much influenced by her father, who ruled the house with an iron fist, was often
absent, and when he was there, he was rageful.

6 Neurological Indicators in Art

There is a confounding factor when trying to understand art developmentally, and that is neurological differences. A significant thread in my practice has been working with people whose brains work differently either by their constitution or because of medical trauma or injury. An art therapist's best practice can be supported by their ability to identify neurological indicators in art. If a patient's art demonstrates that they have neurological involvement, an art therapist will be able to proceed more effectively in both treatment and interventions by being aware of this. If a clinician is aware of a patient having neurological differences, in addition to social, emotional, and behavioral issues, they could ensure better outcomes by structuring treatment more concretely and modifying expectations. Sessions should be structured to allow for optimal benefit for the patient. Patience is essential because goals will be accomplished more slowly due to lack of retention.

Victor, who was discussed in Chapter 3, was engaging in his glue dribbling urethral indulgent play in his art therapy session. As he often did, he shook sparkles over the glue lines which gave them definition. This image appeared which looks like a brain. My sense was that this was an unconscious message revealing that there were some neurological issues which were impacting developmental and behavioral ones.

Although the brain is a vast unexplored region, theories and research have been exponential for decades leading to an expanding understanding of how our brains work and how this affects us. One such category offering insight and explanations is *Neurodiversity*. This is an approach to learning and disability that argues diverse neurological conditions are the result of normal variations in the human genome. Proponents assert that neurological differences should be recognized and respected as a social category. In *Thinking in Pictures* (2006), Grandin describes how people with ASD think differently and gives examples of her envisioning everything but not always in the way that a neurotypical thinker might. She identifies and describes the need to develop the talents in these three basic categories of specialized brains: visual thinkers, music and math thinkers, and verbal logic thinkers, which may exist in varying combinations.

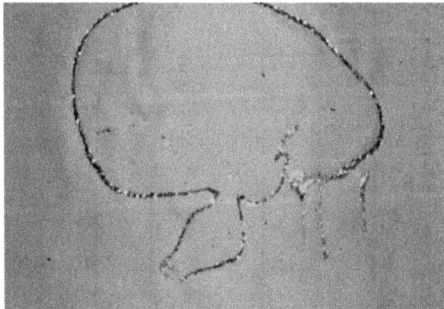

Figure 6.1 Victor's brain

Silver Drawing Test of Cognitive and Creative Skills

A tool that I have found useful for determining if there are neurological issues in patients with whom I work is the *Silver Drawing Test of Cognitive and Creative Skills* (Malchiodi, 2003), copyrighted by Rawley Silver in 1996. Rawley Silver was an art therapist and a cognitive psychologist. The test consists of three components: *Drawing from Imagination, Drawing from Observation, and the Predictive Drawing.*

In the *Drawing from Imagination* part of the test, the tester asks the participant to choose two or more pre-drawn stimulus images and draw something that is happening with interaction between the subjects in these images. When finished, they title the drawing and make up a story. This part of the test assesses emotional content of the participant's responses, their concepts of self and others, and the following cognitive skills: ability to select, combine, and represent.

In the *Drawing from Observation* component of the test, participants are asked to draw an arrangement in a standardized format of three different cylinders and a small stone. This component of the test assesses concepts of space and the ability to represent spatial relationships in height, width, and depth. This component can be useful in both understanding the cognitive level of the participant and seeing if they might have some neurological issues.

The third component of the test is the *Predictive Drawing*. In this component, the participant's ability to sequence is tested, along with their sense of conservation. For example, the participant is shown a full glass of soda and is asked to indicate on other glasses the sequence of the soda being consumed from full to empty. This offers information about their cognitive development and offers insight into neurological issues.

Neurological Indicators in Patient Art

From my observation of artwork by patients with neurological differences, I have compiled a list of neurological indicators:

- Drawings executed with shaky lines
- Chaotic imagery drawn quickly
- Person drawings at a lower level of development from the patient's age
- Unrelated objects in the same composition in disorganized juxtaposition to each other
- Distortions in the representation of the head or the head is crossed out
- Gridded patterns
- Distortions in body representations
- Repetitive representation of numbers and letters
- Ignoring one side of the page
- Images floating above the groundline

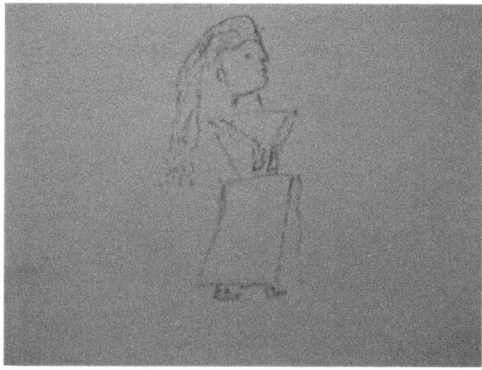

Figure 6.2 Shaky image drawn by a woman who had suffered a stroke

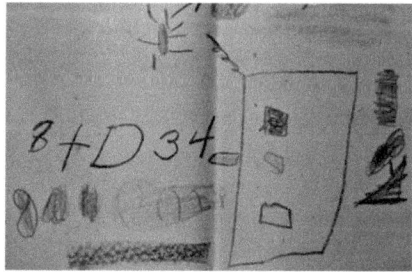 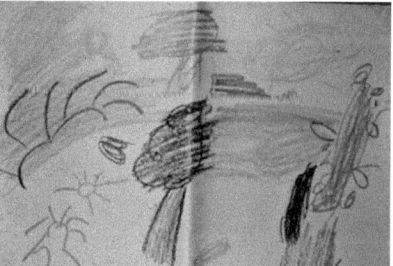

Figure 6.3 Chaotic images drawn quickly, within seconds, by a woman with a severe seizure disorder; she sometimes had 20 seizures in a 24-hour period

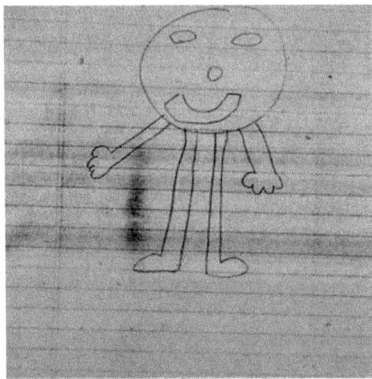

Figure 6.4 Tadpole drawing done by a 16-year-old boy with learning disabilities; it took him over three minutes to complete this simple rendering, which is another indicator of neurological involvement

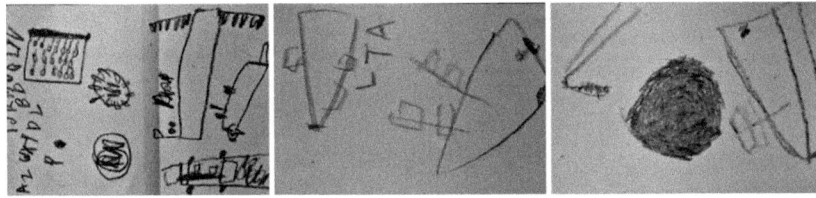

Figures 6.5 Drawings done by adults with neurological developmental disabilities: A plane, cow, and typewriter float in the sky, and a truck is on the ground; A race car and boat float sideways on the page; A shaver, basketball, and ship are all the same size and float on the page

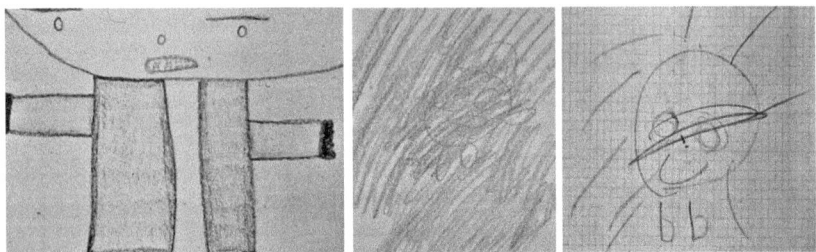

Figures 6.6 Wide open skull drawn by an adolescent who was a sociopath and had developmental disabilities; Two crossed out cephalopod heads drawn by an adult and a child with ASD

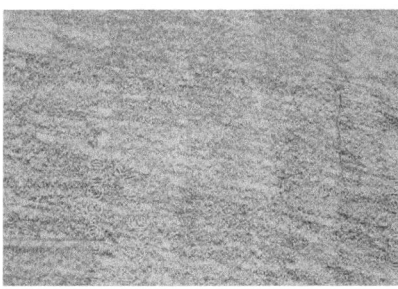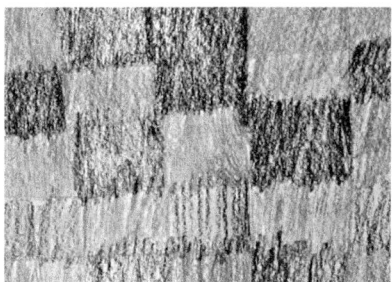

Figures 6.7 Gridded and irregular patterns drawn continuously by a 60-year-old man with Korsakoff's Syndrome from excessive alcoholism; My sense is that he was trying to organize the space to better negotiate it

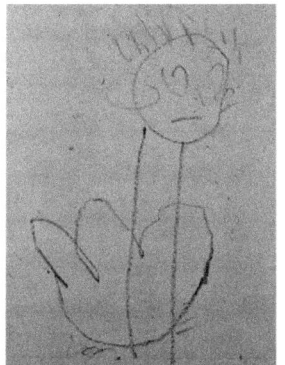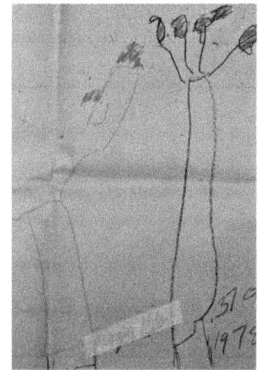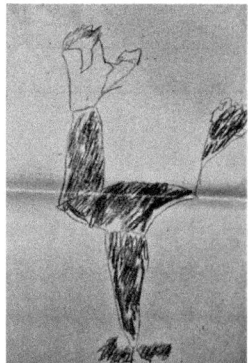

Figures 6.8 Self portrait drawn by a man with developmental disabilities; Two people drawn by a man with cerebral palsy; A person drawn by a woman with dementia

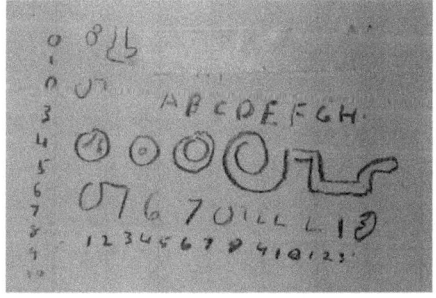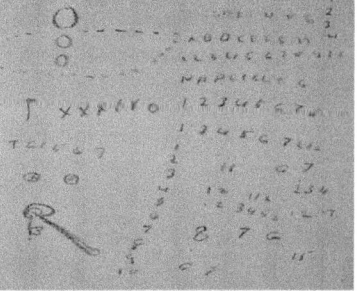

Figures 6.9 Repetitive representation of numbers and letters drawn by a man with neurological impairment from a fever from the Spanish flu at a young age

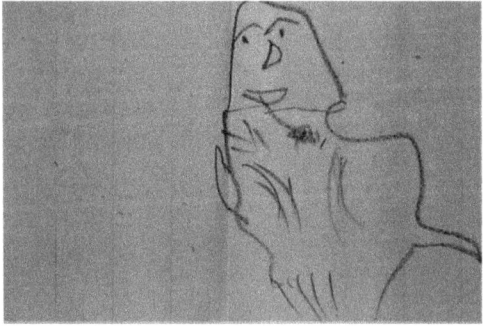

Figure 6.10 A man drawn by a woman who had dementia ignoring one side of
        the page

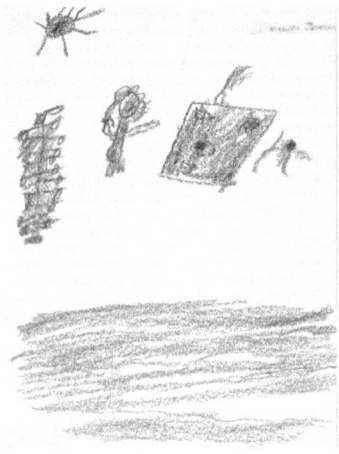

Figure 6.11 A house, tree, and person drawn by a woman who was neurologically
        impaired since birth

Art Therapy Group with ADHD Elementary School Boys

Art therapists need to consider the needs of the group with whom they are
working. Although children with ADHD would willingly use any materials,
it is wise to limit materials and keep them basic. Whether an individual or
group session, I always structure the time very specifically with awareness that
someone with ADHD needs to re-enter the space each time and adjust and
be able to know what to expect. In a group with ADHD elementary aged
boys, the group was very structured to organize and contain participants. For
example, each time they entered the art room, the boys knew where to put
their coats and backpacks, and then they knew to go to the large round table
which I had covered with mural paper. Washable markers were available on

the table, and the boys could draw as we waited for all participants to arrive. Inevitably, the mural became a racetrack as the boys ran around the table enacting the race. Aside from cautioning them not to crash into each other, I was glad that they got some energy out before the group began.

We then each sat in hula hoops, to offer physical boundaries, to check in with each other, and I explained the directive for the day. All the art directives were concrete with few steps to completion. They were focused around knowing themselves better, friends, family, home, school, and community. We did the directive and then returned to a circle to discuss their art. I explained what we would be doing next week. We sang a goodbye song; they put their art in their folders and left. Structure, structure, structure.

7   Family

Timing is everything. I thank the fates that I was still writing this book when the COVID-19 pandemic arrived. Had I been done writing, what I had written about families would have suddenly been obsolete. The world changed overnight, as it never has. With the AIDS epidemic, the world changed, but with the realization of it only being transmitted through contact with a blood-borne pathogen, people knew how to be safe. When there was a terror attack on the World Trade Center in NYC on 9/11/01, the world changed, but as days passed, the world of New Yorkers remained forever changed and got worse. But the rest of the world went on with minimal change in their daily lives.

The COVID-19 pandemic is the most significant event to occur in the modern history of the world. Due to shelter-in-place orders everywhere, people were home with family—good, bad, or otherwise. The entire concept of family changed before our eyes. Baby boomers and Gen Xers with empty nests suddenly had their adult children move back home with them from other countries or states in fear of not being able to get home. A Pew Research Center analysis of Census Bureau data, released September 4, 2020, indicated that 52% of young adults in the USA are living at home with their parents surpassing the record of 48% during the Great Depression (Law, September 21/28, 2020). Adult children moved home, with or without family, so that they could work from home and not be stuck in a city paying high rents. If they moved home with their children, they could get childcare coverage and school help for their kids with live-in grandparents or other siblings. The reverse happened as well. Grandparents have moved into their adult children's home to help with the kids to allow the parents to work and, also to help with virtual schooling. There are many cultures who live as multigenerational families. The pandemic may not have the same impact on these families. But it has certainly affected all families around the world.

I am not a family art therapist nor a marriage and family therapist by my education or credentials. However, all therapists work with families because every patient has a family whose history comes into sessions with them. And when therapists work with a child or adolescent, they must work with the family for optimum outcomes.

Family Art Therapy

Hanna Yaxa Kwiatkowska (1978) wrote the classic art therapy text *Family Therapy and Evaluation through Art* in which she tells the early history of the use of art therapy with families. She describes that the origins were in including families in the psychiatric treatment of people with mental illness. Kwiatkowska discusses the development of family art therapy evaluations, techniques, and treatment interventions. Debra Linesch (1993) in *Art Therapy with Families in Crisis*, expounds on the value of a nonverbal treatment intervention like art therapy for overcoming resistances that arise when working with troubled families. In *Integrative Approaches to Family Art Therapy*, Shirley Riley and Cathy Malchiodi (1994) support the use of a social constructivist approach because it enhances the art therapist's sensitivity to and perception of the worldview of the families they treat and encourages the art therapist to reflect on their own self-referential position.

Kinetic Family Drawing

The *Kinetic Family Drawing* (Burns & Kaufman, 1972) is a projective technique in which the subject is asked to draw a picture of everyone in their family doing something. There are accompanying questions and suggested interpretations. The authors offered this as a tool to understand children and hear what they have to say. Their theoretical framework for interpretations is developmental and Freudian. Their research was based on 12 years of data collection and observations of over 10,000 KFDs gathered from individual patients. The use of an action adds a dynamic element to the drawing.

Some of the interpretations offered by Burns and Kaufman are: Bed=sexual or depressive; Crib=feelings for the baby; Garbage=taking out unwanted stuff; Jump rope=encapsulates, or separates subject from others; Refrigerator=deprivation; Stars=deprivation because they are cold and distant; Stop signs=attempts at impulse control; Lawn mower=person using it is castrating; Vacuum=person using it is powerful and sucking up; Balls=indicate where the power is in the family; "A's" appearing in a composition (the end of a swing set, for example) indicate heavy emphasis on achievement; "X's"=taboo.

Handler and Habenicht (1994) did a thorough review of the literature of the KFD and the research in the areas of reliability, normative findings, cultural influences, and validity. The authors are critical of studies that emphasize single KFD indicators and the use of a single interpretation for each of a series of signs. They also discuss the existence of significant age, race, and culturally related differences in KFD performance and stress the need for more detailed normative data in these areas, emphasizing the need for further research with more sophisticated studies that utilize a more integrative approach to interpretation and is transparent regarding the interpretive approach of the clinician using the KFD technique. One of my professors in graduate studies, Josef Garai, suggested we give the directive: *draw a family doing something.* Leaving out *your family* and *together* may provide more equity. This change in the directive distanced the request from the patient's family of origin and allowed for the patient's own concept and experience of family to be represented. It, therefore, offers insight into the patient's ideas, even fantasies, about their family, environment, and support systems.

While I acknowledge the criticism and support Handler's and Habenicht's recommendations, I have used the KFD throughout my career because it gives the therapist valuable insight into family dynamics. In fact, when I see a child for an initial session, I will give every family member in attendance a clipboard with drawing paper and request a KFD. Parents are usually reluctant to comply but will not say no to the therapist in front of their children. I reassure them that no one expects a masterpiece or is judging them, and I almost always get cooperation. If I do not get cooperation, I have just gotten interesting information about the reluctant family member and how that feeds into family dynamics. When they discuss their KFDs as a family, I am privy to a wealth of information about the dynamics of this family.

In addition to gaining knowledge of the family dynamics, KFDs always include people. It is informative regarding developmental levels to observe how someone draws persons. Other common elements in KFDs are houses and trees. Referring to the *House-Tree-Person test* (HTP manual) (Hammer, 1980) can support gaining diagnostic and personality information about the patient.

Family Drawings

One of the advantages in having every family member do a KFD during the initial session is that you get drawings from people of all ages. As a connoisseur of developmental art, I am getting a sampler platter to view and review with delight. When I review the art, I give thought to the developmental ages of each family member. This will help me negotiate the treatment with the family to the benefit of the child or adolescent in art therapy with me.

The Smith Family

The Smith family came to me for art therapy because Mel, the husband and dad, was having a mid-life crisis and moved out of the house precipitously. They were all in shock, and lots of tears were shed in the session. Joni, the wife and Mom, held back her tears and comforted each of the kids when they cried, being intentionally strong. There is a happy ending because Mel was home within a month, but it cut them deeply because they are such a close and happy family. Every one of them is attractive, smart, good at anything they do, athletic, artistic, and, best of all, kind and loving. I admit that I had to choke back tears during the session.

Joni's KFD shows a tight group, which is the family, enjoying their Friday night pizza tradition. Joni's art is somewhere in the preadolescent range. The family cluster literally is tight in design with lots of color and detail and stands out so obviously in this very empty composition. The feeling I get is that Joni is watching something, that is so dear to her, fade away. Chris, the oldest daughter at 15, draws at a Latency Period level with the sea and sky not meeting. She places herself between her Dad and the source of power, the boat engine. Chris is probably the closest to Mel and was feeling very out of control. Jess, the younger daughter, is 11 and draws right on point for a preadolescent. In her drawing, Mom and the girls are lying on the beach, and Dad and Ron are in the water. They are drawn very lightly. If you look closely, you can see anal denseness in one spot in the water. And if you look even more closely, you can see that there is a person underneath. Jess, most likely, drew the person and did not like how it was coming out, so scratched it out. But it has the eerie feeling of being someone who has drowned. Ron, the youngest is nine, and draws well for his age at a preadolescent level. Every family member touches another. He is at one end and Dad is at the other. Ron looks like he is falling off a cliff, and he is because life as he knows it has abruptly come to a halt. The kids have worried looks on their faces. Mom and Dad smile. Ron has put a line down the page separating Dad from the rest of the family, and Mom is reaching through and grabbing him.

The Jones Family

The Jones family came to me for art therapy because they were very worried about Ellen, who suffered from painful panic attacks and burst out crying often, even a few times during the session. Ellen was 11 and was an honor student, president of the

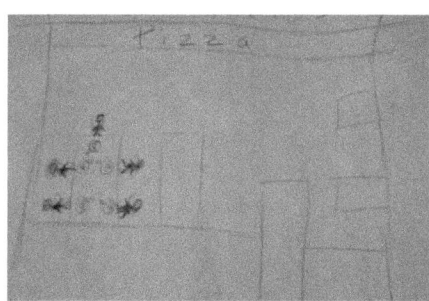

Figure 7.1a Joni's KFD

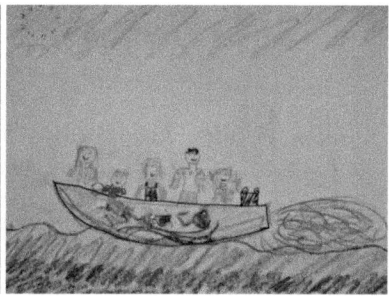

Figure 7.1b Chris's KFD

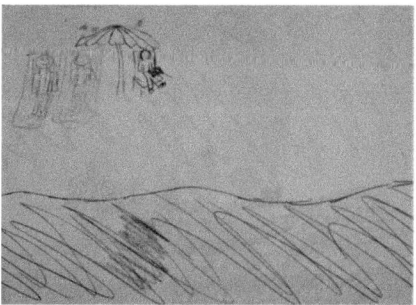

Figure 7.1c Chris's KFD

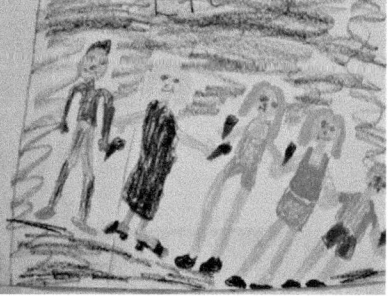

Figure 7.1d Ron's KFD

student council, played sports, and played an instrument. When Ellen was four years old, her brother, Jim, was born. Due to complications at birth, Jim has cerebral palsy with severe cognitive deficits and physical disabilities. The family brought Jim to the session, which indicated an inclusive sense of family, and Ellen went to him often to kiss or hug him. Ellen has completely blocked the time around Jim's birth out of her mind. Ellen's drawing is typically preadolescent with a touch of anime influence. The entire family floats along in the water, almost interconnected, and looking very happy. She reaches for Jim. Because they are in the water, Jim is able to keep up with them as opposed to when he is in a wheelchair. Dad's drawing is in the adolescent range with good representation of perspective and proportion. Mom swings Jim on an adaptive swing, and he and Ellen play ball. There is an obvious connection between them. Mom has them going for a bicycle ride and draws everybody as a stick figure. Mom's drawing is mostly Latency Period, but her representation of foreground and background is adolescent, and she is insightful and can see foreground and background with wisdom. Interestingly, she draws her husband as a little boy. It made me wonder if much of the burden in that family fell on her shoulders.

Individual KFDs

If family is brought up in the conversation during a session with a patient, I may request a KFD. This gives me information that is just not being put into words and gives us some tools to dig more deeply into issues at hand.

Angel

Angel was 14 years old when he entered therapy. He was having depression and anxiety, and his Mom suggested he try therapy. Angel is a good kid and agreed to come. He also likes art and was curious. Angel was a delightful young man, but they lived in a dangerous neighborhood, and his life was stressful. He was very protective of his two younger sisters to the point where he surrendered his new jacket to gang member kids in the neighborhood because they told him they would kill his sister if he did not give them his jacket or if he told anyone who did it. Happily, Angel's parents worked hard to move to the suburbs into a house. Angel was so happy that the first weekend they were there, he rode his bicycle several miles just to say hello to his parents who were at Home Depot.

   Angel's art is typically adolescent. Everyone even has cool foot gear. But Angel has placed himself in the foreground with his hand out as if telling everyone to get behind him. He and Dad look worried. Everyone else looks happy or neutral. And Dad is protecting Mom and baby sister.

Marina

Marina is a 24-year-old Mom of a six-year-old boy with severe disabilities, including being blind and deaf. I asked her to do a KFD. Marina draws at a preadolescent level. In the picture, she, her son, and her boyfriend, who is not her son's father, are

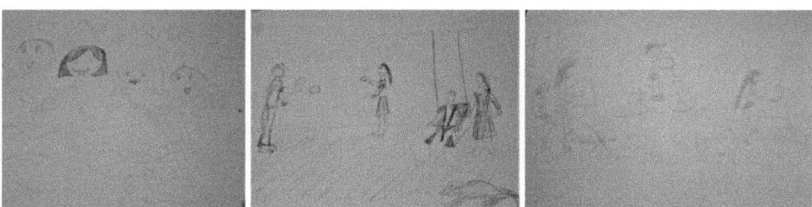

Figure 7.2a–c Ellen's KFD, Dad Jones' KFD, Mom Jones' KFD

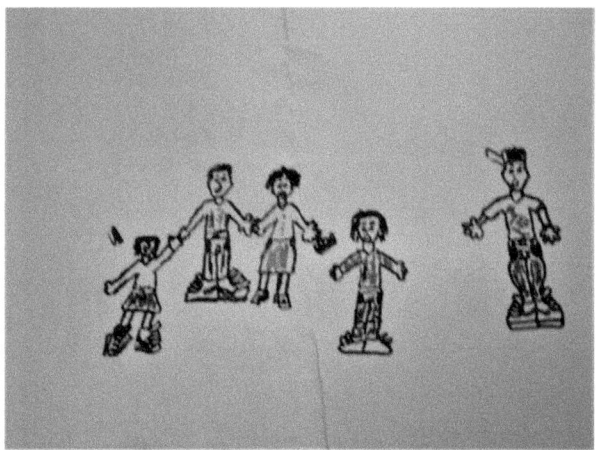

Figure 7.3 Angel's KFD

all huddled in a bean bag chair watching TV. There is an empty feeling to this piece despite cheery windows and smiling faces. Marina gave me more information as she explained the drawing. At her own admission, she is enmeshed with her son and so she is in the picture. Marina goes on to say that, despite his requests, she will not marry her boyfriend, who looks like a little boy here, as she reaches out to him. She will never marry or have another child because she believes that God wants her to only take care of her son. Perhaps that is why there is an empty feeling to this piece.

Mary

Mary is a 22-year-old woman, who lives with her mother. Her mother is narcissistic and constantly reminds Mary about how smart and successful her 29-year-old sister is who does not live at home. When her sister comes home, her mother cooks the fatted calf. Mary is not resentful and loves her sister, and despite all of this, she feels like they are a close family always doing things together. Yet Mary is aware that although she feels close to her mother, she feels like her mother does not feel the same way towards

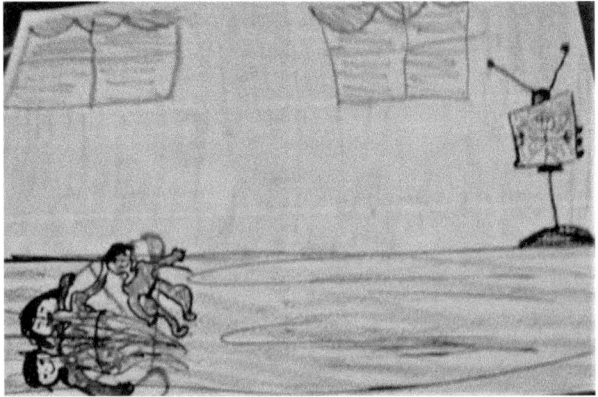

Figure 7.4 Marina's KFD

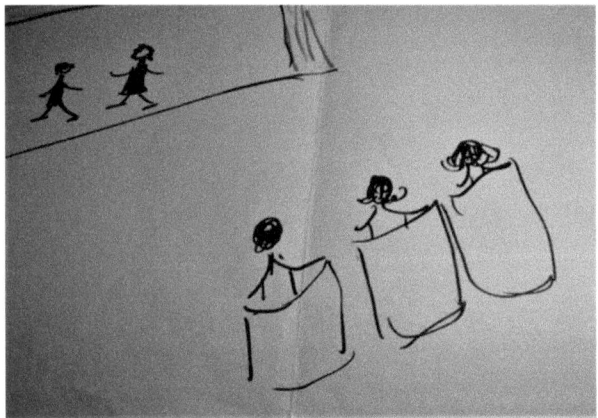

Figure 7.5 Mary's KFD

her. I asked her to do a KFD. Here they are at a Broadway show. Mary's drawings are at a preadolescent level. As we talk about it, it does not occur to Mary that everyone has their back to the viewer. They are not accessible. Mary is at the end, and her mother's and sister's chairs are closer, almost touching. Their arms are visible, but they do not look like they could give good hugs.

Families Around the World

Another aspect of my work on the Board of Advisors for CMA was to participate in curating shows and presentations from their collections. When the museum first opened, CMA placed announcements in art

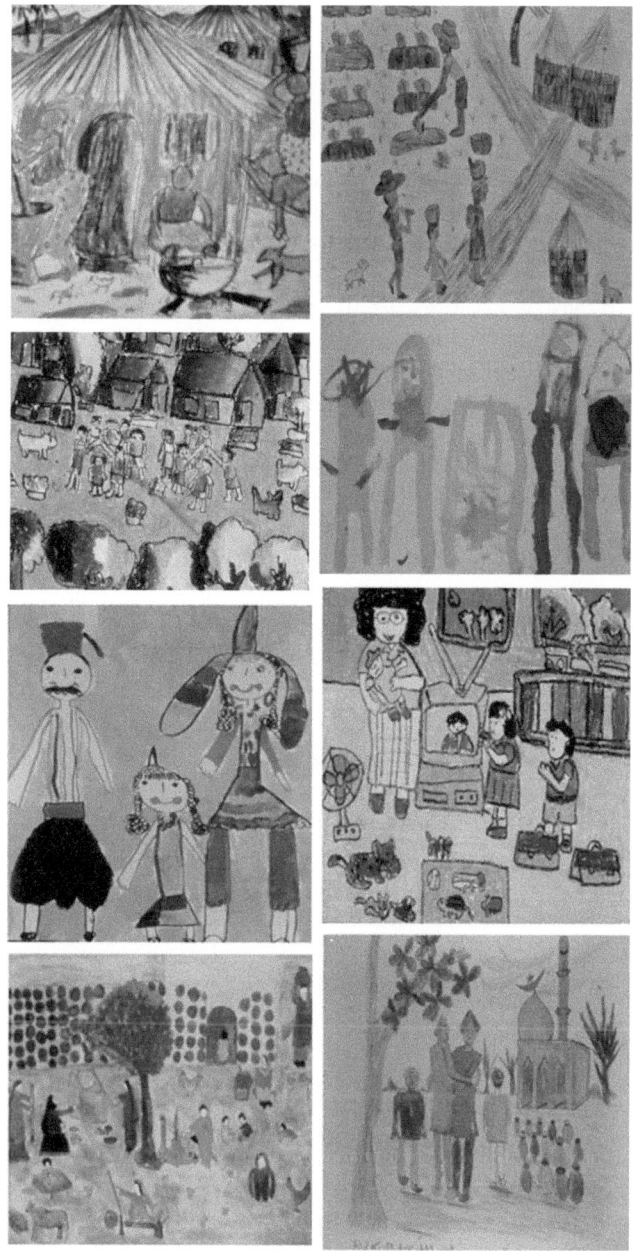

Chart 7.1 Families around the world

education journals internationally requesting the donation of children's and adolescents' art to be displayed and kept in their permanent collection. This exquisite collection had many iterations. At one point, I categorized them thematically to streamline my efforts when preparing presentations for grants or initiatives.

One category is family. The beautiful drawings of families from children and adolescents around the world are joyful to view. There is an aesthetic that transcends the images and creates an exciting visual experience. My assumption is that anyone who submitted art through this *Call for Art* is, most likely, a talented artist. I kept that in mind each time I viewed or reviewed this art. My observations are that formal art training may be a part of the education system in many countries around the world. People whose written language is pictographic have told me that children are exposed to formal art training at a young age because it is essential to their being able to develop writing skills. My personal thoughts are that the art from children from some of these cultures is more stylized and less imaginative. Cultural components are more commonly included in these family drawings than they are in the artwork of children in the USA, including use of color. Other components that are distinct from the art of children from the USA are the use of space and the inclusion of subject matter. My sad interpretation of this is that American children are more wasteful of resources, in general, and may not feel the need to fill all the space on the paper and may simply use more paper.

8 Materials and Techniques Viewed Through a Developmental Lens

The materials and techniques that an art therapist uses in sessions is a very individual decision. My advice to other art therapists is to use whatever materials or techniques with which they are comfortable and familiar. I personally feel that I would not be able to concentrate on the therapeutic needs of my individual patient or patients in a group if I were using a material or technique with which I did not feel at ease. I was doing paper art with an outpatient group of adolescents who had special needs. One of the components of the day's agenda was to make a simple Origami piece. I admitted to the group that I was not that comfortable with the folding, even though I had practiced. Luckily, one of the participants had done Origami in a recreation program. This young man had OCD and applied it to his Origami folding, practicing, and completing intricate patterns. And so, he showed others in the group how to proceed. I was glad to be rescued but felt bad that I was not as well versed in Origami as I should have been when using it in art therapy.

Along these lines, it would be irresponsible to use materials in an environment that is not safe, and so another consideration is the space in which the therapy is done. For example, if an art therapist is a potter, they may have an appropriately equipped studio in which to work with patients using earth clay. A carpeted office is not that space. Moon (2002) says that the studio is where the art therapist is, whether it is at bedside or a nicely appointed art room. This is true, but the art therapist needs to be aware of potential hazards in the environment. The art room on the inpatient behavioral health unit on which I worked had an exhaust fan on all the time. Although it was sometimes an annoying background noise and made it difficult to hear some patients, I always explained to them that it was necessary. We could not open windows and it is essential to have an exhaust system when working with art materials.

Jacobs and Milton (1994) warn art therapists to be aware of the hazards of the materials they use in *The Art of Art Therapy May Be Toxic*. The authors explain public laws that mandate the labeling of hazardous materials and emphasize the responsibility of art therapists in both labeling and informing themselves about potential danger in the use of some materials. The authors described how they took this law quite seriously and made an inventory of their art supplies. They read each label and then either labeled when it had been opened or any hazard warnings. They disposed of some and prioritized other products in terms of their safety when being used with patients. I often discuss the safety of materials with patients, as well as the proper use of same.

Just as I consider developmental levels when assessing a patient, I suggest that art therapists consider a patient's developmental level when choosing materials or techniques. Robbins and Goffia-Girasek, in *The Artist as Therapist*, (edited by A. Robbins, 1987), offer support to my theme of understanding the patient's level of object relations and ego development when offering materials to ensure the holding environment of the art therapy session:

> Using materials in an integrated way with object relations principles becomes an art in itself. Through a developing sense of mastery and familiarity with art materials, an ever-growing repertoire of themes, and a firm developmental grounding, the therapist can determine appropriate usage with a given population or patient.
>
> (pp. 114–115)

There is no doubt that computers have had a huge impact on art and imagery. Many art therapists use computers in their work. I would think computers would be valuable with adolescents who may be resistant to drawing. I must say that I am too old to have the facile use of computers at my fingertips for use in art therapy, but I encourage the use of computers and for art therapists who use them to publish about it.

When I was working in a state hospital early in my practice, I offered tempera paint to a patient who was a regressed and disorganized schizophrenic. By the time I realized my error in judgement, Ralph had covered the paper, the table, and himself with a gooey mess of brown paint which he had mixed from all the colors using his hands. Paint is a material that can cause regression and may be helpful to use if an art therapist wants to support regression in the service of the ego with a patient who is resistant to this and is organized in their thinking. I learned this the hard way and never forgot it. Over time, I have developed a developmental framework to apply to the choice and use of materials and techniques.

The Use of Materials Related to the KAP and Early Childhood

When working with infants and toddlers, I always used a great variety of materials, media, and techniques. But I did observe that some were more applicable to some stages than others and could enhance or support mastery of the phase. For example, children in the urethral indulgent phase enjoyed the flowing quality of watercolor paints and glue. This became a valuable observation to apply to my clinical work because I framed my approach to patients developmentally. If I assessed that a patient had issues originating during their inner genital phase, I would introduce materials and techniques

Table 8.1 KAP Phase-specific materials

Phase	
Oral	Drawing tools—markers, crayons, pencils
Anal	Clays; tempera paints; oil pastels
Urethral	Watercolors; glue; chalk pastels
Inner genital	Reductive sculpture; containers; nesting toys
Outer genital	Additive sculpture; stickers; building toys and supplies, assemblage

relative to this stage into the session. This use of materials would allow the patient to regress to that stage and would stimulate recall of memories and mastery of unresolved issues. The media and materials were usually used on paper.

Safe use of materials is a tenet of art therapy practice. Art materials must always be used in a well-ventilated space. When working with children, waterproof markers should be used and not permanent markers. The latter may be toxic. At CDR, the art therapists would put tape on the back end of pencils, markers, and crayons in case babies put them in their mouths so that they would not ingest any of the material, even if non-toxic. Paints and glues must be non-toxic when used with children. With adolescents and adults, I may use oil paints that require toxic solvents or stronger adhesives, but they are used with precautions and warnings.

Oral: Drawing Tools—Markers, Crayons, Pencils

The baby in the oral stage makes light lines on paper, and basic drawing materials work for this. The baby is not making a strong statement. Interestingly, people with psychosis may prefer basic drawing materials because they often do not want to make a strong statement with their art and may need to maintain a sense of ego integration.

James

James was a 38-year-old man with paranoid schizophrenia. He was agoraphobic, so I worked with him in his mother's home. James was very apprehensive to use any art materials or to make graphic representations. I offered him manilla drawing paper and colored pencils—the manilla drawing paper made the pencil marks seem lighter as opposed to stark white paper. James became less fearful of drawing. When he drew, it was always with light lines on the paper.

James's art contained oral aggressive, urethral indulgent, and urethral aggressive lines. James would tell seemingly nonsensical stories as he drew. I began to connect the symbols that appeared in his drawings with the content of the story. Over time, I realized that he was telling me a story about his being sexually abused by a minister of religion. I used his own symbols and words to let him know that I knew what had happened. James was relieved that I had figured it out and was less anxious and was

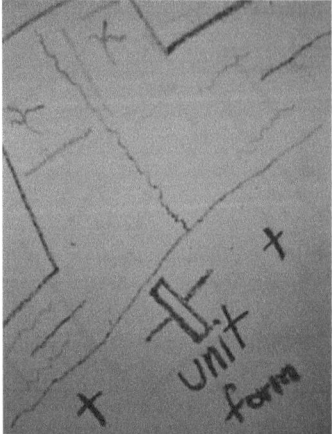

Figure 8.1 James's symbolic communication

able to begin leaving the house for short, very proscribed walks to buy cigarettes and snacks.

Anal: Clays, Tempera, Oil Pastels

Oil pastels are a material that is a bridge between the light drawing of the oral stage and the dense energy of the anal stage. Similarly, the thickness of tempera paints offers that dense artmaking experience. Clays seem obvious materials for the anal stage. The making a mess, pushing, pulling, squishing, and pounding that clay allows are all components of anal play. There are endless varieties of clays from earth clay, which would need to be used in a proper studio, to modeling clays to Model Magic® to Playdoh®. There are many recipes for homemade playdoh which are inexpensive and easy. Some modeling clays are hard to knead and may even leave dye stains on one's hands. Easy-to-knead modeling clays made with colorfast dyes are the best to use in art therapy sessions.

Annie

Annie was an eight-year-old girl who retained her feces. She was very bright and artistically gifted. Her schoolteachers and piano teacher loved her. However, her retaining her feces was becoming a behavioral, social, and emotional problem and was causing her to have some medical problems.

There is a lot to Annie's story of retaining which had to do with both her mother having a series of unsuccessful pregnancies and her father being very controlling. But in the early stages of treatment, I offered user-friendly modeling clay. As Annie kneaded it, she began to pass gas. At first, she tried to pretend it was not happening, but it persisted. Annie looked at me as if to say, "how could you?", but she continued to work the clay. Finally, the anal rhythms took over, and she rushed to the bathroom to have a bowel movement.

Of course, this was not a resolution by any means, but it was a beginning of focusing on the anal issues that were interfering with her daily functioning.

Urethral: Watercolors, Glue, Chalk Pastels

Flowing materials like watercolor paints and glue are urethral stage materials. Just dribbling school glue onto paper is a thrill. Since this type of glue dries clear, color may be added to the glue, or glitter or colored sand may be sprinkled onto the wet glue preserving the design. Water play or use of a sand tray play can also enhance urethral play in sessions. Chalk pastels have a urethral quality because the chalk dust flows, or dusts, away from the surface. Chalk pastels are very toxic to breathe in, so use with children is not advisable.

Bernadette

Bernadette, in her early 30s, was stuck in the anal phase in her body efforts and in her ability to express her feelings and emotions. She had tantrums and became hysterical like a two-year-old; she withheld feelings and affection. Bernadette had been born with part of her colon missing and an unformed anus, therefore needing surgery as a newborn to correct this. Bowel elimination became a daily activity to which she devoted much attention and energy.

Bernadette was married and wanted to have a baby with her husband, with whom she had an unsatisfying sexual relationship. My sense was that neither of them really worked at their sexual relationship. One day, Bernadette drew a picture of the two of them playing in a sandbox and throwing sand at each other. Both looked like little kids, and neither had a face. To me, it epitomized their relationship—immature, little attention to the other's needs, and a kind of facelessness of a poor relationship.

My sense was that she was trying to move out of anal and towards urethral. Sand is a urethral material because of its flow as it runs through fingers and toes. I offered her the sand tray and suggested that she just run her hands and fingers through it for the sensation. Bernadette was almost giddy the first time, joyfully giggling as she played in the sand. She clearly relaxed as she did it, and her tense, anal manner softened. She asked if she could use the sand tray to relax at the start of each session. We soon moved along to her using watercolor paints, and her emotions and behavior seemed to move through the urethral phase and to inner genital. Bernadette became more forthcoming in her communications with her husband. Their relationship improved in many areas including expressing more affection and care for each other and an improved sex life. Bernadette did become pregnant. She, understandably, was fearful of giving birth vaginally because she had early reconstructive surgery and a life of paying attention to every time that she had a bowel movement, and so, her healthy baby was born through a Caesarean section.

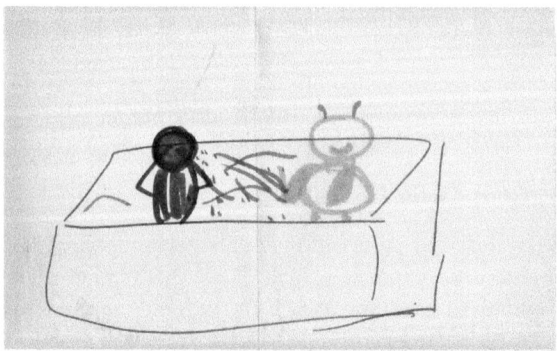

Figure 8.2 Bernadette and her husband in the sandbox

Inner Genital: Reductive Sculpture, Containers

The inner genital stage is when a circle appears. When considering materials and techniques for the inner genital, think about the inner genital child. They are pondering where babies come from and becoming clear about me-not me. In reductive sculpture, there is a carving away to reveal a form previously hidden within, like a birth. Children in this stage love nesting toys, which are containers for each other—like the uterus that they are interested in. They will make art, sign their name (urethral aggressive), fold up the paper, often apply tape and/or staples liberally, place it all into an envelope and deliver it to someone personally. They love bags, boxes, backpacks, or any containers. They will put things into the bag, take things out, carry it with them, and may even want to sleep with it. It is a container for their *babies*. My three-year-old grandson places objects in containers around the house. Months after Christmas, we found the engineer figure from Pa's (my husband) G-gauge Christmas train in a container of petroleum jelly. Of course, in keeping with the inner genital spirit, children of this age often have a doll or stuffed animal that is a constant companion. This is both their baby and a transitional object (Winnicott, 1953) that supports their separation/individuation (Mahler, 1975).

Derek

Derek was a five-year-old boy whose parents were divorcing, which included him moving away from his Dad to a different state. Both his parents were narcissistic and not particularly affectionate. He had a much older sister from his Mom's first marriage, who was protective of him but had her own busy teenage life outside of the home. Derek was anxious and depressed. He played with the nesting toys in my office during each session. Derek often made art that he would put into at least one envelope, securing it with tape. Derek usually left these containers in my care. He would make stories in my sand tray with lots of fighting scenarios and fences and barriers between sides. But each story ended with a baby being buried in the sand for protection. He always asked if I could leave it undisturbed until his next session. Because I could not guarantee that, we would take a photo at the conclusion of the sand tray story and dismantle it. Derek would always leave the buried baby, and I would be careful to return it to the tray before Derek's session if someone else had used the sand tray. We have worked together on many stories, over the years that included rescuing that baby, only to return it to its safe hiding place. This inner genital play helped Derek become his own baby, and his anxiety was reduced as he gave himself the nurturing that his parents had not.

Outer Genital: Additive Sculpture and Stickers, Assemblage

The outer genital stage is mostly known for its aggressive energy. This might translate into punching clay or pounding with a hammer or the use of any material or execution of any technique with gusto. Additive sculpture is a technique related to the outer genital stage and involves hammering or gluing or taping wood or any objects together, or even welding metal together. Of course, the latter technique would require a specific workshop or studio with equipment not readily found in an art therapist's office. Assemblage, which is a process in which a three-dimensional artistic composition is made from putting together found objects, is an outer genital art technique. Building is also outer genital play and can be done with blocks, Legos®, or cardboard tubes. And decorating any three-dimensional art, which is created seems to be a component of phallic art or simply characteristic of four-year-old art. This can be done with stickers, stampers, tape, and markers.

Monty

Monty, an artist who was 39, was trying to resolve his anger towards and painful relationship with his family, as he faced a terminal illness. His parents and brother were all narcissistic and were more concerned with the lucrative family business and material possessions than genuine relationships with each other. They did not understand why Monty wanted to start his own business and move far away from them and did not put any effort into trying to understand. Monty was gay and had AIDS—neither of which they knew about. Monty always assumed that he was unlovable.

Monty was creative, and his art had an inner genital quality in that his designs were forms, which were open containers filled with other forms and lots of color. The inner genital child is pensive, thoughtful, curious, and wise. My sense was that I had to help Monty push through his inner genital phase to his outer genital stage to support his ability to separate from his family and feel whole and individuated. I offered wood, which I imagined he would carve out—reductive sculpture. His response was enthusiastic, and he asked me to bring a few pieces of wood and a hammer and nails. I was pleasantly surprised at his intention to make an additive sculpture, which is outer genital art; just the suggestion to engage in three-dimensional art had jumped Monty out of inner genital into outer genital energy. Monty made a poignant art piece, using family images and cards he had received from his family. The processing of the sculpture enabled Monty's insight into how little his family cared about anyone. He realized that he is not unlovable, rather, they were incapable of love. Monty realized his own self love and embraced his outer genital energy. He faced his terminal illness with grace and tenacity. Ultimately, he told his family but held no expectations regarding their reaction, knowing he was strong and loved himself.

Preschool and School Aged Children

One of the joys of children this age is that they are uninhibited when it comes to art expression and use of materials. They will try and are excited by new techniques. This is one of the reasons that Rubin (1984) calls this stage a time of *Experimenting* and *Consolidating*. If I were to list all the materials recommended for the latency period child, I would probably exceed the word count assigned by my editors. Suffice it to say, anything that is safe, goes.

Students have often teased me that I should be a sales representative for the company *Binney & Smith*, who are the manufacturers of Crayola® brand products. The fact is, they manufacture a variety of quality products and sell them at reasonable prices. Many art therapists work on restricted budgets, so this is valuable information. Interestingly, Jacobs and Milton (1994), when reviewing art materials in terms of their safe use by patients, gave a stamp of approval to *Binney & Smith* products as being safe for patient use. Further, many of the people we treat have limited resources and may not be able to afford costly art supplies. Because I encourage patients to make art outside of the art therapy session, I want to inform them of good values so that they will buy them and use them on their own.

Crayola® manufactures a wide variety of crayons and in different sizes and shapes to fit hands of all ages and flexibility. There are basic colors, sparkle, neon, swirl, and more. They produced multicultural packs so that children would have a range of skin tones when drawing people. While I think this is great, my observations have been that children often do not color in faces of the people they draw. They will color in arms and legs, but it is difficult for younger children to fill in color on the face without covering over the drawn features. Older children have the dexterity and perception to do so.

Markers are loved by children of all ages. There are also many varieties of markers from basic colors to scented to stampers and beyond. Markers are easy to use and are visible on paper which gives the child clear visual feed-back. Tempera and acrylic paints can be offered to children of this age and allow them to experiment with mixing colors.

School glue, stick glue, and rulers are safe to use and enjoyed by children. Because they are in Piaget's *Concrete Operational* stage rulers are a favorite so they can be exacting. Pencils, both regular and colored, are often included in school supplies for children of this age. They will easily use them in making art. And erasers go along with this package because children like to be able to correct mistakes. Again, children should be given good quality #2 pencils and a quality brand of colored pencils. Quality gum erasers and pink erasers are essential tools for children. Poor erasers can smear writing or artwork or not completely erase something, which can be upsetting and frustrating to a young artist.

Children of this age enjoy coloring books. As much as I railed against this as a younger art therapist, observing children of this age using coloring books convinced me that there is a sense of pride by staying in the lines and having a pre-drawn picture that is part of the final product. This would be consistent with Rubin's *Containing Stage*. I have also observed that simple coloring books or posters help people with acute symptoms of psychosis calm down and organize their thinking. And coloring books have come a long way in content and presentation and are available for children and adults.

Preadolescents and Adolescents

As children approach the age at which they might stop drawing and have little interest in artmaking, art therapists must have a deep bag of tricks to engage them. Often, giving them a choice about which materials to use can empower them. But it should be a few choices, not endless opportunities. Novelty markers sometimes attract children of this age. And I cannot say enough about the appeal of stickers and stampers at this age. Offering more sophisticated paints, like watercolors or oil paints may appeal to them because they learn that these require more technical expertise of which they are capable. Sculpture can be done with wood, stone, metal and found objects and allows for three-dimensional representation. Ceramics, using earth clay, kilns, and glazes provides children of this age the opportunity to create a beautiful product, which will enhance self-esteem.

Preadolescents

Keeping it simple works well for everyone. Consistent with this is the benefit of simple craft kits and step-by-step art projects because these give children a strong sense of accomplishment and supports ego development. I worked in a special education junior and senior high school with another art therapist who had worked on a child and adolescent long-term behavioral health unit. Although our budget was meager, he ordered simple model kits for cars and planes and simple leather craft kits. He asked me to trust him and told me he was acting on experience. When the kits arrived, he showed me model cars that could be assembled from as few as five pieces of plastic using school glue, as opposed to toxic modeling glue. There were also wallets that could be easily assembled because they had pre-punched holes, precut lanyard for stringing, and pre-inserted snaps to close the wallet. The next time I ran an art therapy group with six boys with ADHD, ODD, and cognitive deficits, I pulled out the wallet kits. I was glad that I had trusted the other art therapist because every boy in the group sat and completed a wallet to bring home without the usual high energy and sassy talk. They were all so proud at the end of the group, cleaned up, and thanked me for a good group.

Adolescents

Along these lines, the technical arts offer preadolescents and adolescents an avenue of expression that does not necessarily involve being able to draw or paint something representational and results in an aesthetic product. Silk screening, etching, photography and video appeal to preadolescents and adolescents. Being in Piaget's stage of Formal Operations, they can grasp the steps involved in technical arts and explore personal creativity.

Permanent markers are toxic, however, when working with teens in a special education school in NYC, I knew that graffiti was important to them, and they use permanent markers for this process. I did purchase a studio set of Dri-marks® for the kids to use with careful supervision. Of course, I had to count them all and insist that they be back in the rack before anyone could leave the art therapy session. Using art therapy sessions to represent their Tag name in graffiti was invaluable in supporting the kids' development of trust in the process and increase their self-esteem and sense of identity.

More than one co-worker and student has heard me say that if you have sidewalk chalk and bubbles with kids of all ages, you cannot have a bad day. This hypothesis has proven to be true dozens of times throughout my career. I have seen kids with criminal records, with social anxiety, with severe mental illness, and with learning differences participate in chalk walk activities with abandon and joy. Add bubbles, and the mood gets better. Differences and troubles disappear, and adolescents become like little kids playing together. Sometimes the latency period child emerges as they might cooperate towards a theme. Sometimes the adolescent child emerges as they might decide to represent a political or social statement. Thankfully, instant photography allows art therapists to capture the image. This can be a teaching moment to help them understand that not everything is permanent, and one can learn to let go. I explain to them the sand art tradition of indigenous people. This tradition calls for creating art with sand, which then blows away. The belief is that the winds take away some issues from the maker of the art, and what is left behind is for the maker to ponder and resolve.

Chalk Walk

Although most of my chalk walk experiences have been great and productive fun, there was one that caused problems. I always tell the kids that they cannot use offensive symbols or words. This is important for publicly displayed art, and they are compliant. One day, I took the adolescents from the behavioral health unit outside to play with chalk and bubbles. We all had a good time, and the kids were well-behaved, and these good spirits lasted for the rest of the afternoon. They were all very cooperative and forthcoming in art therapy groups for the rest of the day. When we returned to the unit, the nurse manager greeted us at the door and asked to speak to me. She had received an angry call. It seems that a visitor to the hospital had complained to administration that the kids were drawing symbols that were racist and offensive. I was confused and asked what the problem was, assuring my boss that I did not think this to be the case. She informed me that the visitor felt that a six-pointed star that looked like the Star of David was anti-Semitic. My initial reaction was great annoyance because I know that many kids draw stars that way because it is easier than making a typical five-pointed star, but I also recognized that my boss had been reprimanded by the administration and was unhappy with me. I apologized to her and then said, "I am sorry that you *had to be yelled at by administration, but this was the most normal thing these kids have done for days." She knew that one of my war cries was to treat adolescents with respect and with as much "normalcy" as possible. Her mood softened and she listened to me but asked that I never do this again. I agreed but was sad that an art experience that was so valuable had to be deleted from my repertoire.*

Adults

As I have repeated often, most adults are resistant to making art. Sometimes, they refuse. I will usually explain that they do not have to be an artist to be in art therapy and that I have an expanded concept of creativity. I might point their creativity out to them. For example, I recently had a discussion with a patient, Shana, who did not want to draw and was adamant that she is not artistic or creative. I told her that I thought her cooking was creative which made her take notice. I mentioned that she started almost every session by reporting about some dishes she had made and how she might have changed something here or there because she did not have an ingredient or wanted to use something she already had. Shana loved to share her food with friends and neighbors and was prideful when they liked it. While she is still resistant to artmaking, I feel it is important to acknowledge personal creativity and empower patients to use that creativity to improve their lives.

For simplicity and for their comfort, I offer adult patients basic markers and 9″ × 12″ drawing paper on a clipboard during an individual session. It often stays on the couch next to them. In fact, I had a 20-year-old patient who very obviously pushed the markers and clipboard away from her as she sat down on the couch each week. But even resistant patients may be willing to draw something if these supplies are readily available and easy to use. If something comes up that they are having trouble explaining with words, I will suggest they try to draw it. They are usually relieved when I accept their drawing with no criticism and are, then, engaged as we process it together.

Because adults are reluctant to draw, photography can be used. And collage goes easily with photography. Cutting and pasting photographic and magazine images and creating a collage is relatively easy and satisfying. Because there is no expectation of rendering a representational drawing or painting, the patient has the freedom to combine images to express themselves.

Linda

Linda had gone through a difficult divorce and continued to raise her children without her ex-husband's help. He had done things to humiliate her and was behind on child support. Linda had grown through therapy and by taking charge of her own life and was doing well. But she had lingering anger towards her ex-husband that she felt was interfering with her potential. I suggested that she bring in copies of her wedding pictures and scout around for other meaningful images to bring in as well and explained that she could make a collage. Linda made a collage using and altering these images. She added comments with markers. She made her ex-husband look like a devil, and she made herself look like a superhero. The process was very cathartic for Linda, and she giggled freely as she got deeper into it, remarking that this was one of the best art therapy sessions she had had.

Color

There are many opinions on color and how it is used in art therapy. I personally feel that color used in art therapy is very subjective. Color choice is very culture and trend driven. Consider the TV show *Orange is the New Black* to understand my point. When I was a little girl, my great aunt, who was from Puerto Rico showed me her wedding shawl. It was black silk with beautifully embroidered red and pink flowers all over it. She told me that Spanish brides wear black, but many other cultures wear white as a wedding color. And in the next breath she made it clear to me that I was too young to wear black and should not do so until I was eighteen. One of the only identified color uses with which I agree is if an adolescent uses the combination of black and red, it could be an indicator of suicidal ideations.

Some of the color theories certainly have validation and can inform art therapy practice. Hammer (1980) discusses the color symbolism of the *House-Tree-Person* (HTP) test stating that although there is empirical data suggesting that certain colors indicate certain feelings or emotions, he warns that it is not always so hard and fast. However, Hammer indicates that with the use of color, that is, the chromatic HTP, as opposed to the achromatic HTP, "…the clinician is provided with an instrument which taps a deeper personality" (Hammer, 1980, p. 234). In the *Art Therapy Sourcebook,* Malchiodi (2007) provides a chart of *Common Color Associations* with the caveat that it is intended to stimulate thoughts about colors and what their personal meaning might be to the art therapist but points out that colors may have contradictory or ambiguous meaning. The example she offers is the color red because it is associated with both love and anger. And in *Understanding Children's Drawings,* Malchiodi (1998) reminds art therapists that color has different significance depending on the child's level of development. For example, younger children tend to choose colors that have an emotional meaning to them, so they will draw someone they like with a color they like, latency period children will be very concrete in their use of color, and adolescents may be more interpretive in their use of color.

9 Epilogue

This is a picture of my office with 46 years of research and patients' notes and artwork all over the room. As hard as it is to believe, I know where everything is because I am a great believer in organized chaos. My husband is always shocked when I ask him what he was looking for on my desk because, to him, it looked like a mess. But I know where everything is, or was, if it had not been disrupted by my husband looking for something! I am a bit grateful for the pandemic because I have not had to clean up my office for patients in between working on the book. I see most of my patients by Zoom and have re-purposed a small room in my house and dragged in my *grab-and-go* box of traveling art supplies so that I may see the few patients who come in person in that room.

I have been poring over all of this for several months. With each artwork viewed or session note read, I wrote something in my head or jotted a quick note on the folder. Always a teacher, I intended to write about *all* of it and impart my wisdom and experience to others so they may learn from it. My head swirled with different iterations of how I would present all, yes all, of this. I felt like Superman in the capsule coming to Earth from Krypton. And I was in that capsule for 46 years. Throughout Superman's journey, the voice of his father, Jor-El, spoke imparting all the knowledge of Krypton, so that his son could carry it on after the cataclysmic destruction of their planet. But I was not in a capsule coming from Krypton, I was in my office on a fast track to becoming mad. I prayed that my dear editors, Amanda Devine and Gabrielle Vernachio, would not open this manuscript to find hundreds of pages filled with the run-on sentence, "All work and no play makes Beth a dull girl," not unlike the sentence that Wendy Torrance found on pages and pages next to Jack's typewriter in *The Shining*. If you are reading this, I guess my work makes sense.

One day while rocking my new grandson, the swirling in my head seemed to start to gel. It occurred to me that I can write another book or some articles and talk about other aspects of my research. I did not have to get it all down in one book. And what was gelling galvanized. What I saw was my hypothesis about understanding art developmentally, and the research that would support this got in line with my hypothesis. My book title, which was Amanda's idea, is *Applying Developmental Art Theory in Art Therapy Treatment*

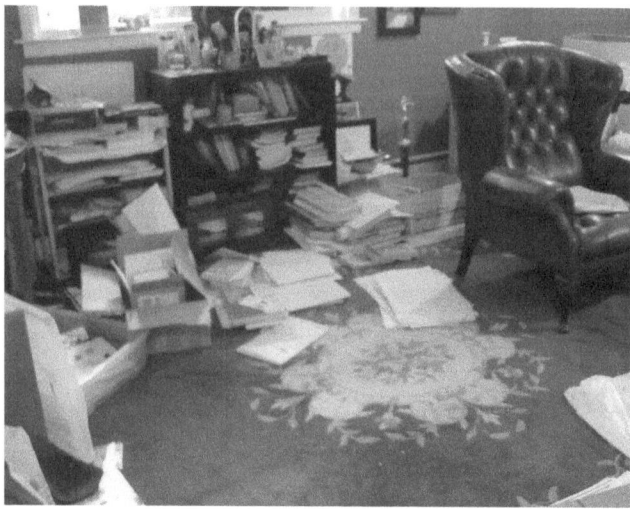

Figure 9.1 Step into my office

and Interventions: Illustrative Examples through the Life Cycle. This is exactly what I wanted to convey. For decades, I taught child art therapy, which obviously included developmental theory. And I always structured it to focus on looking at developmental indicators in the artwork of patients of all ages. But the course also included assessments and clinical topics in which I did not necessarily have expertise, but I honed up so that I could teach it well and usually brought in an art therapist who worked in that field of practice. None of this needed to be in this book. I was not writing an inclusive textbook. I was writing on my hypothesis with my research. Anything other than that could be put aside for now.

As I said in the introduction, this is my life's work—*my* life's work. Human development and the artwork that rises out of each stage from womb to tomb fascinates me. That passion is obvious in my presentation of my work. I have tried to make my hypothesis as clear as possible by organizing the chapters to be relevant and informative.

Object relations informs my practice, and I have explained its relevance to the creative arts therapies. It is my great pleasure to finally publish the Kestenberg Art Profile, with the blessing of Dr. Kestenberg's daughter, Janet Kestenberg Amighi. My hope is that the KAP will offer creative arts therapists a developmental lens with which to view patient art, thus giving them a window into the patient's developmental history and an opportunity to make effective and supportive interventions. I have also reviewed theories of human development, per Freud, Piaget, and Erikson, and developmental art theory per DiLeo, Gardner, Kellogg, Kestenberg, Levick, Lowenfeld, and

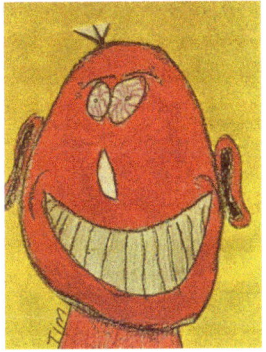

Figure 9.2 Self portrait of a genius

Rubin. These have been paired with illustrative cases to make the information clearer.

The next chapter is devoted to trauma. We live in a traumatized society, a traumatized world. Every patient whom creative arts therapists treat has experienced some level of trauma in their lives and understanding developmental components of this can support best practice. Another significant thread in my experience has been working with people with neurological differences, and I have observed that this can be seen in their art and impacts interventions, choice of materials, goals, and outcomes.

Families are part of human development, so I have included information and research to support creative arts therapists as they negotiate the intricacies of working with families. Of course, working with families means developing sensitivity to culture and ethnicity, and I have addressed this when appropriate but strongly encourage creative arts therapists to inform themselves on these matters for their patients.

Art materials, media, and techniques are the tools of the trade for art therapists. I have included a chapter on materials, media, and techniques and frame their use from a developmental perspective.

My work on the Board of Advisors with the Children's Museum of the Arts in SoHo, NYC, was ten of the most satisfying years of my career. Through this experience, I became familiar with the art of children and adolescents living through war and refugeeism. Through my affiliation with the museum, I was able to give back to my community by developing and implementing several programs after the terrorist attacks on the World Trade Center on 9/11/01 for two years. Finally, as a member of the Board of Advisors I had access to the museum's permanent collection of international children's and adolescents' art. I learned from this artwork, taught about it to students, and organized it into presentations for school administrators and grant proposals. And I can think of no better way to end this book than showing my favorite piece from the international collection. The piece is entitled *Self Portrait of a Genius* by a 12-year-old boy named Tim. Every time I look at it, I am filled with joy, laugh out loud, appreciate kids' art, think that I feel like he looks, and wonder what Tim is doing right now. So, Tim, wherever you are, you really are a genius.

References

Andruk, S. (1996). Earthquake! *Art Therapy: Journal of the American Art Therapy Association, 13*(2), 136–140.

Avrahami, D. (2006). Visual art therapy's unique contribution in the treatment of post-traumatic stress disorders. *Journal of Trauma & Dissociation, 6*(4), 5–38.

Baird, K. & Kracen, A.C. (2006). Vicarious traumatization and secondary traumatic stress: A research synthesis. *Counselling Psychology Quarterly, 19*(2), 181–188.

Baker, B. (2006). Art speaks in healing survivors of war. *Journal of Aggression, Maltreatment, & Trauma, 12*(1–2), 183–198.

Bergman, A. (1978). From mother to the world outside: The use of space during the separation- individuation phase. *Between reality and fantasy: Transitional objects and phenomena.* New York, NY: Jason Aronson Press.

Boenig, P. (1976). *Awakening: A rebirth through images* (Unpublished master's thesis) Pratt Institute, Brooklyn, NY.

Bornstein, M.H. (1975). Qualities of color vision in infancy. *Journal of Experimental Child Psychology, 19*(3), 401–419.

Buday, K.M. (2013). Engage, empower, and enlighten: Art therapy and image making in hospice care. *Progress in Palliative Care, 21*(2), 83–88.

Burns, R.C. & Kaufman, S.H. (1972). *Action, styles, and symbols in kinetic family drawings: KFD.* New York, NY: Routledge.

Chang, I.I. (2005). Theatre as therapy, therapy as theatre transforming the memories and trauma of the 21 September 1999 earthquake in Taiwan. *Research in Drama Education: The Journal of Applied Theatre and Performance, 10*(3), 285–301.

Deri, S. (1978). Transitional phenomena: Vicissitudes of symbolization and creativity. *Between reality and fantasy: Transitional objects and phenomena.* New York, NY: Jason Aronson Press.

DiLeo, J. H. (1970). *Young children and their drawings.* New York, NY: Brunner/Mazel.

DiLeo, J. H. (1973). *Children's drawings as diagnostic aids.* New York, NY: Brunner/Mazel.

DiLeo, J. H. (1977). *Child development: Analysis and synthesis.* New York, NY: Brunner/Mazel.

DiLeo, J. H. (1983). *Interpreting children's drawings.* New York, NY: Brunner/Mazel.

Eigen, M. (1980). On the significance of the face. *Psychoanalytic Review, 67*(4), 425–439.

Erikson, E.H. (1950). *Childhood and society.* New York, NY: Norton.

Feen-Calligan, H. (2007). The use of art therapy in detoxification from chemical addiction. *Canadian Art Therapy Association Journal, 20*(1), 16–28.

Feen-Calligan, H., McIntyre, B., & Sands-Goldstein, M. (2009). Art therapy applications of dolls in grief recovery, identity, and community service. *Art Therapy: Journal of the American Art Therapy Association, 26*(4), 167–173.

Feil, N. (1993). *The validation breakthrough: Simple techniques for communicating with people with "Alzheimer's-type dementia."* Baltimore, MD: Health Professions Press.

Freud, A. (1937). *The ego and the mechanisms of defense.* London: Karnac Books.

Freud, A. (1944). Sex in childhood. *Journal of the American Psychoanalytic Association, 2*(1), 2–6.

Freud, A. (1963). The concept of developmental lines. *The Psychoanalytic Study of the Child, 18*(1), 245–265.

Freud, A. (1969). Adolescence as a developmental disturbance, 5–10. In G. Caplan & S. Lebovici (Eds.), *Adolescence: Psychosocial perspectives.* New York, NY: Basic Books.

Freud, S. (1905). *Three essays on the theory of sexuality* (SE VII) (pp. 145–243). London: Hogarth.

Freud, S. (1923). The ego and the id. *The standard edition of the complete psychological works of Sigmund Freud, 19.* London: Hogarth Press.

Gardner, H. (1980). *Artful scribbles: The significance of children's drawings.* New York, NY: Perseus.

Goldhahn, E. (2011). The pleasure of finding: A perspective on acts of finding in movement and in visual art informed by object relations theory. *Body, Movement and Dance in Psychotherapy, 6*(1), 69–76.

Gonzalez-Dolginko, B. (2002). In the shadows of terror: A community neighboring the World Trade Center disaster uses art therapy to process trauma. *Art Therapy: Journal of the American Art Therapy Association, 19*(3), 120–122.

Gonzalez-Dolginko, B. (2003). Art therapists are increasingly dealing with trauma: Let's make sure we're all prepared. *Art Therapy: Journal of the American Art Therapy Association, 20*(2), 106–109.

Gonzalez-Dolginko, B. (2016). Picture of health: An artist's journey through disease as told in his photographs. *Journal of Applied Arts & Health, 7*(3), 369–389.

Grandin, T. (2006). *Thinking in pictures: My life with autism.* New York, NY: Vintage.

Haeseler, M.P. (1987). Censorship or intervention: "But you said we could draw whatever we wanted!" *The American Journal of Art Therapy, 26*(1), 11–20.

Hammer, E.F. (1980). *The clinical applications of projective drawings* (6th ed.). Springfield, IL: Charles C. Thomas.

Handler, L. & Habenicht, D. (1994). The kinetic family drawing technique: A review of the literature. *Journal of Personality Assessment, 62*(3), 440–464.

Hastie, S.C. (2006). The Kestenberg Movement Profile. *Creative arts therapy manual* (pp. 121–132). Springfield, IL: Charles C. Thomas.

Heegaard, M. *They draw out your feelings series.* Minneapolis, MN: Woodland Press.

Horay, B. (2006). Moving towards gray: Art therapy and ambivalence in substance abuse treatment. *Art Therapy: Journal of the American Art Therapy Association, 23*(1), 14–22.

Horner, A. (1979). *Object relations and the developing ego in therapy.* New York, NY: Jason Aronson.

Jacobs, J. & Milton, I. (1994). The art of art therapy may be toxic. *Journal of the American Art Therapy Association, 11*(4), 271–277.

Jones, J.G. (1997). Art therapy with a community of survivors. *Art Therapy: Journal of the American Art Therapy Association, 14*(2), 89–94.

Kellogg, R. (1967). *Analyzing children's art.* Palo Alto, CA: National Press Books.

Kestenberg, J.S. (1967). *The role of movement patterns in development.* New York, NY: Dance Notation Bureau Press.

Kestenberg, J.S. (1968). Outside and inside, male and female. *Journal of the American Psychoanalytic Association, 16*(3), 457–520.

Kestenberg, J.S., Marcus, H., Robbins, E., Berlowe, J., & Buelte, A. (1971). Development of the young child as expressed through bodily movement I. *Journal of the American Psychoanalytic Association, 19*(4), 746–764.

Kestenberg, J.S. & Sossin K.M. (1979). *The role of movement patterns in development 2.* New York, NY: Dance Notation Bureau.

Kestenberg Amighi, J., Loman, S., Lewis, P., & Sossin, M. (1999). *The meaning of movement: developmental and clinical perspectives of the Kestenberg Movement Profile.* New York, NY: Routledge.

Kestenberg Amighi, J., Loman, S., Sossin, K.M. (2018). *The meaning of movement: Embodied developmental, clinical and cultural perspectives of the Kestenberg Movement Profile* (2nd ed.). New York, NY: Routledge.

Klein, M. (1957). *Envy and gratitude: A study of unconscious sources.* London: Tavistock Publications.

Kübler-Ross, E. (1969). *On death and dying.* New York, NY: Simon & Schuster/ Touchstone.

Kübler-Ross, E. & Kessler, D. (2005). *On grief and grieving: Finding the meaning of grief through the five stages of loss.* New York, NY: Scribner.

Kwiatkowska, H.Y. (1978). *Family therapy and evaluation through art.* Springfield, IL: Charles C. Thomas.

Laban, R. (1966). *The language of movement: A guidebook to choreutics.* Boston, MA: Plays.

Landy, R.J, (1994). *Drama therapy: Concepts, theories, and practice* (2nd ed.). Springfield, IL: Charles C. Thomas.

Langer, S. (1954). *Philosophy in a new key: A study in the symbolism of reason, rite, and art.* (6th ed.). Cambridge: New American Library.

Law, T. (2020). How many young adults moved home amid the pandemic? *Time.* New York, NY: Time USA.

Levick, M. (1998). *See what I'm saying: What children tell us through their art.* Dubuque, IA: Islewest.

Linesch, D. (1993). *Art therapy with families in crisis.* New York, NY: Brunner/Mazel.

Lobban, J. (2014). The invisible wound: Veterans' art therapy. *International Journal of Art Therapy, 19*(1), 3–18.

Loman, S. & Brandt, R. (1992). *The body mind connection in human movement analysis.* Keene, NH: Antioch New England Graduate School.

Loman, S. & Foley, L. (1996). Models for understanding the nonverbal process in relationships. *The Arts in Psychotherapy, 23*(4), 341–350.

Lowenfeld, V. (1987). Therapeutic aspects of art education. *The American Journal of Art Therapy, 25,* 111–146.

Lowenfeld, V. & Brittain, W.L. (1957). *Creative and mental growth* (3rd ed.). New York, NY: Macmillan.

Luquet, G.H. (1913). *Les Dessins d'un enfant: Étude psychologique.* Paris: Librairie Felix Alcan.

Mahler, M. (1968). *On human symbiosis and the vicissitudes of individuation.* New York, NY: International Universities Press.

Mahler, M.S., Pine, F., & Bergman, A. (1975). *The psychological birth of the human infant: Symbiosis and individuation.* New York, NY: Basic Books.

Malchiodi, C. (1998). *Understanding children's drawings.* New York, NY: Guilford Press.

Malchiodi, C. (2003). *Handbook of art therapy.* New York, NY: Guilford Press.

Malchiodi, C. (2007). *The art therapy sourcebook.* New York, NY: McGraw Hill Professional.

Mitchell, J. (Ed.) (1986). *The Selected Melanie Klein.* New York, NY: Free Press.

Moon, C. (2002). *Studio art therapy: Cultivating the artist identity in the art therapist.* Philadelphia, PA: Jessica Kingsley.

Moos, R. & Timko, C. (2008). Outcome research on twelve-step and other self-help programs. In M. Galanter & H. O. Kleber (Eds.), *Textbook of substance abuse treatment* (4th ed.)(pp. 511–521). Washington, DC: American Psychiatric Press.

Naff, K. (2014). A framework for treating cumulative trauma with art therapy. *Art Therapy: Journal of the American Art Therapy Association, 31*(2), 79–86.

Nainis, N. (2005). Art therapy with an oncology care team. *Art Therapy: Journal of the American Art Therapy Association, 22*(3), 150–154.

Nainis, N., Paice, J. A., Ratner, J., Wirth, J. H., Lai, J., & Shott, S. (2006). Relieving symptoms in cancer: Innovative use of art therapy. *Journal of Pain and Symptom Management, 31* (2), 162–169.

Nishida, M. & Strobino, J. (2005). Art therapy with a hemodialysis patient: A case analysis. *Art Therapy: Journal of the American Art Therapy Association, 22*(4), 221–26.

Obernbreit, R. (1985). Object relations theory and the language of art tools for treatment of the borderline patient. *Art Therapy: Journal of the American Art Therapy Association, 2*(1), 11–18.

Ogden, P., Pain, C., & Fisher, J. (2006). A sensorimotor approach to the treatment of trauma and dissociation. *Psychiatric Clinics of North America, 29*, 263–279.

Piaget, J. (1936). *Origins of intelligence in the child.* London: Routledge & Kegan Paul.

Piaget, J. (1973). Intellectual evolution from adolescence to adulthood. *Readings in Child Psychology.* New York, NY: Appleton-Century-Crofts.

Piaget, J. & Inhelder, B. (1948). *Representation of space by the child.* Paris: Presses Universitaires de France.

Riley, S. (1996). Reauthoring the dominant narrative of our profession. *Art Therapy: Journal of the American Art Therapy Association, 13*(4), 289–292.

Riley, S. & Malchiodi, C. (1996). *Integrative approaches to family art therapy.* Chicago, IL: Magnolia Street Publishers.

Robbins, A. (Ed.). (1987). *The artist as therapist.* New York, NY: Human Sciences Press.

Robbins, A. (1989). *The psychoaesthetic experience: An approach to depth-oriented Treatment.* New York, NY: Human Sciences Press.

Robbins, A. & Goffia-Girasek, D. (1987). In A. Robbins (Ed.), *The Artist as Therapist* (pp. 104–115). New York, NY: Human Sciences Press.

Roje, J. (1995). LA '94 earthquake in the eyes of children: Art therapy with elementary school children who were victims of disaster. *Art Therapy: Journal of the American Art Therapy Association, 12*(4), 237–243.

Room, R. & Greenfield, T. (1993). Alcoholics anonymous, other 12-step movements and psychotherapy in the US population. *Addiction, 88*(4), 555–562.

Rothbaum, B.O., Meadows, E.A., Resick, P., Foy, D.W., Foa, E.B., Keane, T. M., Friedman, M. J. (Eds.). (2000). *Effective treatments for PTSD: Practice guidelines from the International Society for Traumatic Stress Studies.* New York, NY: Guilford Press.

Rothschild, B. (2000). *The body remembers: The psychophysiology of trauma and trauma treatment.* New York, NY: W.W. Norton.

Rubin, J. (1984). *Child art therapy* (2nd ed.). New York, NY: Van Nostrand Reinhold.

Rubin, J. (ed.). (1987). *Approaches to art therapy: Theory and technique.* New York, NY: Brunner/Mazel.

Schilder, P. & Wechsler, D. (1935). What do children know about the interior of the body? *International Journal of Psycho-Analysis, 16*, 355–360.

Searles, H.F. (1960). *The nonhuman environment.* New York, NY: International Universities Press.

Searles, H.F. (1979). *Countertransference and related subjects: Selected papers.* New York, NY: International Universities Press.

Silver, R. (1979). *Developing cognitive and creative skills through art: Programs for children with communication disorders or learning disabilities.* Mamaroneck, NY: Albin Press.

Skeffington, P.M. & Browne, M. (2014). Art therapy, trauma and substance misuse: Using imagery to explore a difficult past with a complex client. *International Journal of Art Therapy, 19*(3), 114–121.

Spitz, R.A. (1955). The primal cavity: A contribution to the genesis of perception and its role for psychoanalytic theory. *The Psychoanalytic Study of the Child, 10*(1), 215–240.

Terr, L. (1991). Childhood traumas: An outline and overview. *American Journal of Psychiatry, 148*(1), 10–20.

Van der Kolk, B., McFarlane, A., & Weisaeth, L. (Eds.). (1996). *Traumatic stress: The overwhelming experience on mind, body and society.* New York, NY: Guilford Press.

Wadeson, H. (2003). Art as therapy for Parkinson's disease. *Art Therapy: Journal of the American Art Therapy Association, 20*(1), 35–38.

Waller, C. (1992). Art therapy with adult female incest survivors. *Art Therapy: Journal of the American Art Therapy Association, 9*(3), 135–138.

Winnicott, D.W. (1953). Transitional objects and transitional phenomena—a study of the first not-me possession. *The International Journal of Psychoanalysis, 34*, 89–97.

Winnicott, D.W. (1965). *The maturational process and the facilitating environment.* New York, NY: International Universities Press.

Winnicott, D.W. (1971a). *Playing and reality.* London: Routledge.

Winnicott, D.W. (1971b). *Therapeutic consultations in child psychiatry.* New York, NY: Basic Books.

Zammit, C. (2001). The art of healing: A journey through cancer: Implications for art therapy. *Art Therapy: Journal of the American Art Therapy Association, 18*(1), 27–36.

Index